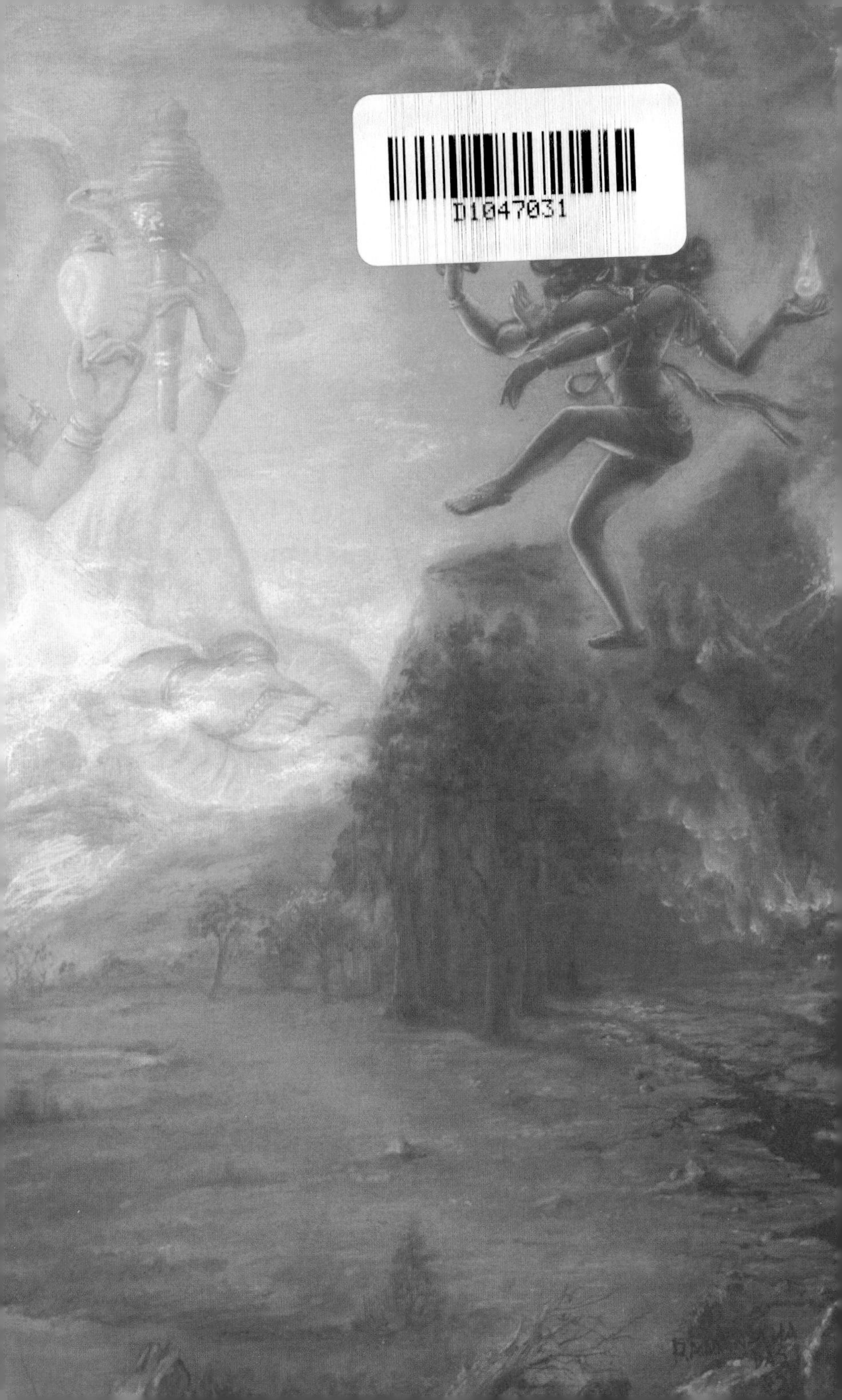

The QUEST for ENLIGHTENMENT

BOOKS by
His Divine Grace A. C. Bhaktivedanta Swami Prabhupāda

Bhagavad-gītā As It Is
Śrīmad-Bhāgavatam (18 vols.; with disciples)
Śrī Caitanya-caritāmṛta (9 vols.)
The Nectar of Devotion
Kṛṣṇa, The Supreme Personality of Godhead
Teachings of Lord Caitanya
Śrī Īśopaniṣad
The Nectar of Instruction
Easy Journey to Other Planets
Kṛṣṇa Consciousness: The Topmost Yoga System
Perfect Questions, Perfect Answers
Teachings of Lord Kapila, the Son of Devahūti
Transcendental Teachings of Prahlāda Mahārāja
Dialectic Spiritualism—A Vedic View of Western Philosophy
Teachings of Queen Kuntī
Kṛṣṇa, the Reservoir of Pleasure
The Science of Self-Realization
The Path of Perfection
Search for Liberation
Life Comes from Life
The Perfection of Yoga
Beyond Birth and Death
On the Way to Kṛṣṇa
Rāja-vidyā: The King of Knowledge
Elevation to Kṛṣṇa Consciousness
Kṛṣṇa Consciousness: The Matchless Gift
The Nārada-bhakti-sūtra (with disciples)
The Mukunda-mālā-stotra (with disciples)
A Second Chance
The Journey of Self-Discovery
The Laws of Nature
Renunciation Through Wisdom
Geetār-gan (Bengali)
Vairāgya-vidyā (Bengali)
Buddhi-yoga (Bengali)
Bhakti-ratna-boli (Bengali)
Back to Godhead magazine (founder)

A complete catalog is available upon request

The Bhaktivedanta Book Trust
3764 Watseka Avenue
Los Angeles, CA 90034, USA
Telephone: 1-800-927-4152
http://www.harekrishna.com/~ara/
E-mail: letters@harekrishna.com

The QUEST for ENLIGHTENMENT

Articles from
Back to Godhead magazine

HIS DIVINE GRACE
A.C. BHAKTIVEDANTA SWAMI PRABHUPĀDA
Founder-*Ācārya* of the International Society for Krishna Consciousness

THE BHAKTIVEDANTA BOOK TRUST
Los Angeles • London • Stockholm • Bombay • Sydney • Hong Kong

ENDPAPERS: The material universe is governed by three deities under the supervision of Lord Kṛṣṇa, the Supreme Personality of Godhead. Lord Brahmā (left) oversees the mode of passion and is entrusted with creation. Lord Viṣṇu (center), a plenary expansion of Kṛṣṇa, oversees the mode of goodness and takes charge of maintenance. And Lord Śiva oversees the mode of ignorance and is the primary agent of destruction.

Readers interested in the subject matter of this book are invited by the International Society for Krishna Consciousness to correspond with its secretary.

International Society for Krishna Consciousness
P.O. Box 34074
Los Angeles, California 90034
USA

Telephone: 1-800-927-4152
http://www.harekrishna.com
e-mail: letters@harekrishna.com

Design: Arcita dāsa
Lord Kṛṣṇa in circle: from a painting by Rāmadāsa-Abhirāma dāsa and Dhṛti-devī dāsī
Lord Brahmā on lotus: from a painting by Rāmanātha dāsa

First Printing, 1997: 55,000
Second Printing, 1998: 50,000
Third Printing, 1999: 50,000
Fourth Printing, 2001: 57,500

Printed in Australia

Library of Congress Cataloging-in-Publication Data

A. C. Bhaktivedanta Swami Prabhupāda, 1896-1977
The quest for enlightenment : articles from Back to godhead magazine / A. C. Bhaktivedanta Swami Prabhupāda.
p. cm.
ISBN 0-89213-292-2
1. Yoga. Bhakti. 2. Yoga. I. Title.
BL 1238.56.B53A33 1997
294.5'512—dc21 97—41422
CIP

CONTENTS

Introduction

Many people are reacting to today's high-pressure, fast-paced life by "downshifting." They accept lower incomes to pursue their special interests or to live with less stress in more natural surroundings. Often they will devote more time and energy to spiritual pursuits. Instead of vacationing in Disneyland, they explore the mysteries of Stonehenge, Egypt's pyramids, or the temples of the Maya in southern Mexico. They find more inspiration and illumination in the teachings of lost civilizations than in the offerings of our modern consumer society. Surveys of students routinely report an increasing interest in spiritual fulfillment.

This is a healthy trend. The sages of ancient India said, *tamasi mā jyotir gama*—"Don't stay in darkness, go toward the light." They advised thoughtful people to embark on the quest for enlightenment. The final goal of this quest is not, however, attained by everyone. The *Bhagavad-gītā,* India's classic book of spirituality, informs us that out of thousands of people who set out on the quest for enlightenment only a few will take to the right path, and of those who find the right path, only the most fortunate will achieve the final goal. Spiritual success requires determination and perseverance.

It also requires understanding the difference between matter and spirit, darkness and light. Today such understanding is rarely found, even among spiritual seekers. The *Gītā* informs us, "What is night for all beings is the time of awakening for the self-controlled; and the time of awakening for all beings is night for the introspective sage." In his commentary on this passage in his *Bhagavad-gītā As It Is*, His Divine Grace A. C. Bhaktivedanta Swami Prabhupāda (known popularly as Śrīla Prabhupāda) says, "Activities of the introspective sage . . . are night for persons materially absorbed.

Materialistic persons are asleep in such a night due to their ignorance of self-realization. The introspective sage remains alert in the 'night' of the materialistic men. The sage feels transcendental pleasure in the gradual advancement of spiritual culture, whereas the man in materialistic activities, being asleep to self-realization, dreams of varieties of sense pleasure, feeling sometimes happy and sometimes distressed in his sleeping condition."

In this book, *The Quest for Enlightenment*, Śrīla Prabhupāda shows us the true path of enlightenment and invites us to traverse this path from the dark night of materialism to the shining daylight of transcendence. Widely recognized by scholars and spiritual leaders as the most distinguished teacher of Indian culture and philosophy in the modern age, Śrīla Prabhupāda is the perfect guide and companion for the journey along the path of enlightenment.

The Quest for Enlightenment is a compilation of Śrīla Prabhupāda's teachings, originally published as articles in *Back to Godhead,* the magazine of the Hare Kṛṣṇa movement. Śrīla Prabhupāda founded this magazine in India in 1944, and since then it has become the world's foremost journal dedicated to the teachings of Lord Kṛṣṇa.

The first chapter of this book describes the need to embark on the quest for enlightenment. The second explains what matter is, what spirit is, and who controls them both. In the third chapter we learn about the attributes of the best kind of spiritual master to guide us on our personal quest. The fourth chapter outlines the techniques of yoga and meditation, and the fifth chapter explores spiritual solutions to material problems. In the sixth chapter Śrīla Prabhupāda critiques modern science and philosophy. And in the seventh and final chapter Śrīla Prabhupāda explains love of God, the highest goal for those on the path of transcendence.

The Quest for Enlightenment provides a comprehensive and comprehensible guide to the path of spiritual progress. Śrīla Prabhupāda speaks the truth without compromise. He represents the Vedic tradition faithfully and without personal motivation. And through his unique gift he communicates the most essential Vedic teachings to the modern world, inviting us all to embark on the journey that will take us from darkness to light, from the unreal to the real, from death to immortality.

The Publishers

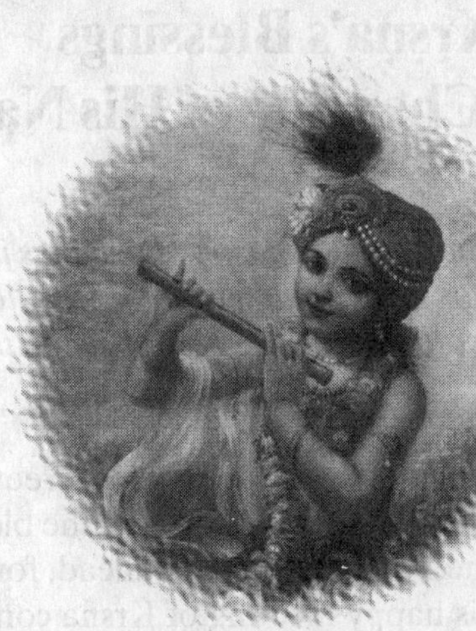

1.
The Quest For Enlightenment

Kṛṣṇa's Blessings In the Chanting of His Name

January 1, 1969. The Hare Kṛṣṇa movement has just arrived in Great Britain, and a gathering of Londoners interested in the movement listens to this message recorded for them by Śrīla Prabhupāda.

Ladies and gentlemen: Please accept my greetings for the happy new year of 1969, and please accept the blessings of Śrī Kṛṣṇa, the Supreme Personality of Godhead, for your kindly participating in this happy meeting of Kṛṣṇa consciousness.

Lord Kṛṣṇa appeared on earth five thousand years ago and gave us the unique philosophy and religious principles of Kṛṣṇa consciousness in the shape of the *Bhagavad-gītā*. Unfortunately, in the course of time, because things change and deteriorate in the material world, people deteriorated and forgot the art of Kṛṣṇa consciousness. Therefore Lord Kṛṣṇa again appeared as Śrī Caitanya Mahāprabhu* at the end of the fifteenth century to revive the same Kṛṣṇa conscious atmosphere in human society.

Lord Caitanya's special gift to the fallen souls of the present Age of Quarrel and Disagreement is to induce people in general—religionists, philosophers, everyone—to take to the chanting of the holy name of Kṛṣṇa. Lord Caitanya informed us that the Absolute Supreme Personality of Godhead can descend in transcendental sound and that when we chant the Hare Kṛṣṇa *mantra* offenselessly we immediately contact Kṛṣṇa in His internal energy. Thus we immediately become purified from all the dirty things in our heart.

Our conditioned life of material existence is due to dirty things in our heart. Originally we are all Kṛṣṇa conscious liv-

*Śrī Caitanya Mahāprabhu is Lord Kṛṣṇa Himself. He appeared five hundred years ago in Bengal, India, and taught love of God through the congregational chanting of His holy name.

ing beings, but because of our long association with matter, we have been transmigrating from one form of body to another, suffering in the cycle of birth and death in various species of life (numbering 8,400,000). Every one of us, although originally a spiritual soul and therefore qualitatively one in constitution with the Supreme Lord, Kṛṣṇa, has identified with our material body. Thus we are being subjected to various material pangs, headed by birth, old age, disease, and death.

The whole material civilization is a hard struggle against birth, old age, disease, and death. Against these perpetual problems human society is struggling fruitlessly in many ways. Some people are making material attempts, and some are making partially spiritual attempts. The materialists are trying to solve the problems through scientific knowledge, education, philosophy, ethics, literature, and so on. The salvationists are trying to solve the problems by putting forth various ways of discerning matter from spirit. And some people are trying to overcome birth and death through mystic yoga.

But all of these people—the materialists, the salvationists. and the yogis—must know it for certain that in this Age of Kali, the Age of Quarrel and Dissension, there is no possibility of success without accepting the process of Kṛṣṇa consciousness.

Śrīla Śukadeva Gosvāmī, the speaker of the *Śrīmad-Bhāgavatam,* has therefore recommended that whether you are a fruitive worker, a salvationist, or a mystic yogi, if you actually want to be freed from the pangs of material existence you must take to the process of chanting Hare Kṛṣṇa, Hare Kṛṣṇa, Kṛṣṇa Kṛṣṇa, Hare Hare/ Hare Rāma, Hare Rāma, Rāma Rāma, Hare Hare.

Kṛṣṇa consciousness is the art of purifying our heart of the dust of material desires. As living entities we have desire as a component part of our constitution. Therefore we cannot stop desiring. But we can *purify* our desire. Killing desire is no solution, but *curing* desire—the diseased condition of desire—is the right solution. And when the dust of misunderstanding is cleared from our heart, we can see our real position and make steady progress toward the ultimate goal of life.

We have forgotten that the ultimate goal of our life is to revive our lost relationship with God, or Kṛṣṇa. To revive that relationship we should execute all of our activities in Kṛṣṇa consciousness. We do not ask you to cease your present occupational duties; we simply recommend that you execute those duties in Kṛṣṇa consciousness .

Lord Śrī Caitanya Mahāprabhu never recommended that one change his position in life. Rather, He favored the process of staying in one's position and hearing about Kṛṣṇa from a bona fide source. To arrive at the real goal of life, one should give up the artificial process of philosophical speculation and instead submissively hear about the philosophy of Kṛṣṇa consciousness, which is contained in Vedic literatures such as the *Bhagavad-gītā* and *Śrīmad-Bhāgavatam.* If one submissively chants the *mahā-mantra* (Hare Kṛṣṇa, Hare Kṛṣṇa) and hears without any misinterpretation the message of Kṛṣṇa as it is given in the *Bhagavad-gītā,* then one does not have to change his position by some artificial method. Simply by chanting and hearing about Kṛṣṇa you will come to the transcendental position, in which you can know God—His name, His form, His qualities, His pastimes, His paraphernalia, and so on.

We are, however, misled at present by leaders who have very little connection with God, or Kṛṣṇa. Some of them deny the existence of God. Some of them try to put themselves in God's place. Some of them, utterly hopeless and frustrated at being unable to reach any right conclusion, think the ultimate goal of life is void, or zero. But Kṛṣṇa consciousness is solid ground for understanding God directly by the simple method of chanting His holy name.

Misled by spiritually blind leaders, people in general, who themselves are spiritually blind, have failed to achieve their desired success. But here is a method, Kṛṣṇa consciousness, that is directly offered by Kṛṣṇa. He plainly gave us His instructions five thousand years ago in the *Bhagavad-gītā,* and He confirmed them five hundred years ago in the form of Lord Caitanya.

So the Kṛṣṇa consciousness movement is a great art of life, very easy and sublime. The Kṛṣṇa consciousness movement gives you everything you want, without any artificial endeavor. It is transcendentally colorful and full of transcendental pleasure. We prosecute Kṛṣṇa consciousness through singing, dancing, eating, and hearing philosophy received through the authorized disciplic succession of spiritual masters coming down from Kṛṣṇa Himself. Therefore Kṛṣṇa consciousness gives us complete spiritual success, without our undergoing any artificial change of our natural instincts.

Consciousness is already in you, but it is now dirty consciousness. What we have to do now is cleanse our consciousness of all dirty things and make it pure consciousness—Kṛṣṇa consciousness. And we can easily do this by the pleasant method of chanting the glorious holy name of God: Hare Kṛṣṇa, Hare Kṛṣṇa, Kṛṣṇa Kṛṣṇa, Hare Hare/ Hare Rāma, Hare Rāma, Rāma Rāma, Hare Hare.

Understanding the Soul

When it comes to perceiving the soul, hearing—*not seeing—is the way. As Śrīla Prabhupāda declares in this conversation with disciples that took place in Mumbai, India, in April 1977, "You have to get your perception of the soul by hearing from the bona fide spiritual authorities. That is knowledge. Otherwise, who has seen the soul with these paltry eyes?"*

Disciple: Śrīla Prabhupāda, when we try to show people that they're spiritual beings, it's awfully hard for them to see. And when we explain how the soul transmigrates from one lifetime to the next, from one body to the next—sometimes it's next to impossible for people to see.

Śrīla Prabhupāda: Yes. Transmigration—how can it be shown? How can it be seen by the naked eye? Even the mind, intelligence, and ego you cannot see; although they are material, they are so subtle that you cannot see them. And what to speak of the soul?

Still, there *is* a way to perceive these things. For instance, though you cannot see my mind directly, you can see its activities. In this way you can see my mind. Therefore you have to accept its existence. And though with these limited material senses you cannot see my soul, or spiritual form, still you can see my soul acting in so many ways. Therefore you have to accept the existence of my soul.

Another example: All around you here, you have the sky, the ethereal element, but you cannot see it. So where is the proof that the ethereal element exists? [*Claps.*] *That* you cannot see with your eyes. But you can hear it with your ears. *Śabda,* sounds—sound is the proof of the existence of the ethereal element. You cannot see the ether, but it is there.

Sound is the proof for the presence of the ethereal element. And to prove the presence of the soul—which is much, much more subtle than the ethereal element—again you must rely on sound. You need to hear from spiritually realized persons and authoritative scriptures.

Disciple: So with these limited material senses we can perceive the soul only indirectly?

Śrīla Prabhupāda: That's all. To perceive the soul—which is far, far beyond your perceptive power—you need the *śruti,* the authoritative scriptures. *Śruti* means "what is heard"—from the Lord and from spiritually realized sages who know about the existence beyond matter.

So you have to get your perception of the soul by hearing from the bona fide spiritual authorities. That is knowledge. Otherwise, who has seen the soul with these paltry eyes? These modern rascals—who among them has seen the soul? They are educated so grossly.

But everything can be perceived. Not that everything has to be seen with these eyes. We often give this example: as a new-born infant, you cannot determine who is your father simply by your eyes. You have to hear your mother reassuring you, "Here is your father." That's all. You cannot make some experiment through your seeing power. You simply have to hear from your mother, the bona fide authority, on the subject of who is your father. You have to hear. That's the proof. And the proof of the soul's existence is *śruti,* what you hear from the spiritually realized authorities.

Disciple: Śrīla Prabhupāda, wouldn't another proof be that everyone can, say, look at his hands and recall years earlier, when he had the hands of a baby or a young child? So everyone can figure out, "Now that my body is so totally different, my feeling of still being the same person has to be coming from my soul." In other words, what stays the same is your soul.

Śrīla Prabhupāda: Yes. And here is yet another example. You cannot see scent, but still, you know whether the scent is nice or not very nice. Let us say a rose scent is being carried by a breeze. You cannot see the rose scent or how it is being carried. But you can smell it and know without a doubt, "Ah, this is a rose scent."

Similarly, the soul is being carried along through this material world on the subtle breeze of his materially conditioned mind and intelligence and his false ego, his misidentification with matter. But you cannot see the soul directly. You have to learn to see the soul by hearing from the authorities, such as Lord Kṛṣṇa. *Apareyam itas tv anyāṁ prakṛtiṁ viddhi me parām:* "Beyond this material nature, there is another *prakṛti,* another nature." That is the spiritual nature, in which *na jāyate mriyate vā*—"There is no birth or death."

But at present the soul, who is a tiny spark of that undying spiritual nature, is being carried along by his materially covered mind and intelligence, and by his false ego. Now, when our gross material eyes see his body cremated, we may mistakenly think that he is finished, that everything, including the soul, is finished.

The atheists will talk like this. *Bhasmī-bhūtasya dehasya kutaḥ punar āgamano bhavet:* Once your present body is burnt to ashes, where is the question of your having come from a previous life or of your going to a next life? You are finished.

The atheists will talk like this, but Kṛṣṇa does not talk like this. No. He says, *na hanyate hanyamāne śarīre:* "Even when the material body is destroyed, the soul cannot be destroyed."

So whom will you follow—the atheists? Why not follow Kṛṣṇa? That is our proposal.

The atheists will say, "Just see. The body has been burnt to ashes. There—where is the person? The person is dead?"

Kṛṣṇa says, "No, he is not dead. He has gone on to another body." And *dhīras tatra na muhyati:* "Those who are sober are not disturbed by the outward show of the body's death. They know that the soul who lived within has gone to his next life." The real person is still living. He has simply gone from one dwelling place to another.

But who can understand this fact? Only the sober, Kṛṣṇa says. We have to become sober, cool-headed, and mature.

Take the example of a restless child. Now, how can you convince this restless child about higher philosophy, the science of the soul? It is not possible. But a sober person, a cool-headed person—he can be convinced. So this is a childish civilization. It is not a sober civilization.

We have to become sober, spiritually intelligent, cool-headed—not over-identifying with the outer body and restlessly rushing about, driven by bodily whims. But these so-called modern men—these restless rascals—have built their whole civilization on rushing about and being driven by bodily whims. Now, how will they become sober and cool-headed?

The only hope is for them to take advantage of this Kṛṣṇa consciousness movement.

The You That Doesn't Change

Consciousness is the essence of all life. A chief subject for study in our schools, one would think. "Unfortunately," Śrīla Prabhupāda says in this talk given in April, 1968, at Boston University's Marsh Chapel, "the modern educational system has no department for teaching about consciousness or the spirit soul, although this knowledge is the most important."

Kṛṣṇa consciousness, the science of God, is very important because it enables us to understand God and our relationship with Him. Of course, in every religion there is some conception of God: "God is great." But simply understanding that God is great is not sufficient. We must have knowledge about our relationship with God.

Generally, we take it for granted that God is our order-supplier. So those who believe in God usually approach Him in distress or when they're in need of money. Then there are some who approach God out of curiosity, and a few who want to understand the science of God. These are the four classes of men who are interested in God, and they all have a background of pious activities. Without a background of pious activities, a person will not be interested in the science of God. Therefore those who are unfortunate, who are impelled by impious activities, do not believe in God; they never care for God. So it is very difficult for the atheists to understand God.

Still, because Kṛṣṇa consciousness is a science, even an atheist can appreciate it if he is intelligent. Atheist or theist, everyone is conscious. That is a fact. It doesn't matter whether you believe in God or you do not believe in God: you are conscious. As soon as I pinch any part of your body, you at once protest, "Somebody is pinching me! I am feeling pain!" Even in the animals there is consciousness.

Now, what is this consciousness? The *Bhagavad-gītā* says, *avināśi tu tad viddhi yena sarvam idaṁ tatam:* "Consciousness is that which is spread all over your body, and it is eternal."

How is consciousness eternal? That you can understand by practical experience. In your childhood you were conscious, in your boyhood you were conscious, in your youth you were conscious, and as you progress to old age you will be conscious. So your body is changing, but your consciousness continues unchanged. This you cannot deny. Therefore the *Bhagavad-gītā* says, *na hanyate hanyamāne śarīre:* "Consciousness is eternal. It is not vanquished with the destruction of the temporary body."

As soon as there is no consciousness in the body, the body is dead. Then what is consciousness? It is the symptom of the presence of the soul. Just as a fire situated in one place distributes heat and light everywhere, the spirit soul present in your body spreads consciousness all over your body. This is a fact.

From your childhood body to your boyhood body to your youthful body, your consciousness continues. Similarly, your consciousness will carry you into another body, and that transmigration from one body to another is called death. When your old body cannot be maintained anymore, the consciousness has to be transferred to a new body. When your garment is too old, it has to be changed. Similarly. when the material body is too old to carry on, your consciousness is transferred to another body and you begin another life. This is the law of nature.

But unfortunately the modern educational system has no department for teaching about consciousness or the spirit soul, although this knowledge is the most important. Without consciousness, without the soul's being present, the body is useless. Unfortunately, we take very good care of the body but have no knowledge of consciousness or the spirit soul. This ignorance is due to *māyā,* or illusion. We are very serious about the nonpermanent things—the body and its extensions, which will not exist, which will be vanquished after a certain period of years—but we do not care about the eternal consciousness, the spirit soul, which is transmigrating from one body to another. Ignorance of the spirit soul is the main defect of modern civilization.

As long as we are unaware of the presence of the spirit soul in the body, as long as we do not inquire about the spirit soul, all our activities are simply a waste of time. This is stated in the *Śrīmad-Bhāgavatam* [5.5.5]: *parābhavas tāvad abodha-jāto yāvan na jijñāsata ātma-tattvam.* Anyone who has accepted a temporary body is understood to be foolish. So every one of us is born foolish, because we identify ourselves with the temporary body. Everyone knows that his body will one day not exist, but everyone still identifies himself with his body. This is ignorance, or illusion.

Nearly everyone in the world is immersed in this ignorance, for they do not know that they are spirit souls transmigrating from one body to another. Although no one wants to die, cruel death is forced upon everyone. But people do not consider this problem very seriously. They think they are very happy following the principles of animal life—eating, sleeping, mating, and defending. At the present moment people are very proud of the advancement of human civilization, but they are almost totally concerned with these four principles. According to the Vedic literature, this way of life is no better than the animals'.

Human life is meant for advanced knowledge. And what is that advanced knowledge? To know oneself, to answer the question, What am I? In every civilized society there is some set of religious principles, whether Islam or Christianity or Judaism or Hinduism or Buddhism. And what is the purpose of the scriptures and religious principles? To understand consciousness, to understand the spirit soul and how it has fallen into material, conditioned life, how it is transmigrating among various species of life, and how it can be released from this cycle of birth and death. There are 8,400,000 species of life, and we have been wandering among them since time immemorial. Only when we reach the human form of life do we have the opportunity to ask the question, What am I? If we do not understand what we are, then we miss the opportunity of human life. We simply waste our time in the propensities of animal life—eating, sleeping, mating, and defending.

We must inquire, "I do not wish to die; why is death forced upon me? I do not want to be diseased; why is disease forced upon me?" But even if a person becomes very ill, he will generally not inquire like this. He will simply think, "All right, I am diseased. Let me go to the doctor and get some medicine." But from the innermost part of his heart he doesn't ever want to be diseased, he doesn't want to be dead. Why? Because he is eternal. His real position is eternal life, blissful life, without any death, without any birth, without any disease. So he is missing the opportunity of human life unless he inquires into how he can attain this position.

The human form of life is the opportunity to achieve the highest perfection. If we do not make progress toward that vision, we are simply spoiling this opportunity of civilized human life. I especially mention civilized human life, with developed consciousness, developed education. At this developed stage we should ask, "Why are calamities being forced upon me?" Nobody wants to meet calamities. In every city of your country I see the fire brigade and the ambulance always rushing in the street. Who wants his house to be set on fire? Who wants to meet an accident? These things are being forced on us, but still no one asks, "I do not want these calamities. Why are they being forced upon me?" As soon as we become inquisitive to know why all these miserable conditions of life are being forced upon us, that is the beginning of our self-realization.

Now you are trying to solve these problems through so-called scientific research or so-called philosophical research, but the actual solution is to reform or purify your consciousness. If you purify your consciousness, you will end the process of transmigration from body to body. Of course, now you may be very happy that you have a nice American body. You are enjoying life. But do you know what your next life will be? That you do not know. But you should know that life is a continuity. This present life is only a flash—a moment in our journey through millions of species of life. So the Kṛṣṇa consciousness movement is the movement for purifying consciousness, ending transmigration, and solving all problems.

Kṛṣṇa consciousness is very simple. Simply chant these sixteen words: Hare Kṛṣṇa, Hare Kṛṣṇa, Kṛṣṇa Kṛṣṇa, Hare Hare/ Hare Rāma, Hare Rāma, Rāma Rāma, Hare Hare. We are simply requesting you to chant these sixteen words. There is no loss on your part, but there is immense gain. Why don't you make an experiment? It is not very difficult. Throughout the world thousands are chanting. Although the *mantra* is written in Sanskrit, it is a universal transcendental vibration.

If we take to chanting this *mantra,* we come directly in touch with the Supreme Lord. That makes us purified. If we go near the fire we become warm. Similarly, if we come directly in touch with the Supreme Spirit, our purification begins. So if you chant this Hare Kṛṣṇa, Hare Kṛṣṇa, your impure consciousness will be purified and you will know what you are.

Chanting Hare Kṛṣṇa is the process of cleansing the mind of all dirty things. And as soon as you are cleansed of all dirty things, your material anxieties are over. That is stated in the *Bhagavad-gītā* [18.54]:

brahma-bhūtaḥ prasannātmā na śocati na kāṅkṣati
samaḥ sarveṣu bhūteṣu mad-bhaktiṁ labhate parām

The word *brahma-bhūta* means that as soon as you come to the platform of spiritual understanding, you immediately become joyful and are freed from all material anxieties. You no longer hanker after any profit, nor are you very sorry when there is a great loss (*na śocati na kāṅkṣati*). Then you can see everyone on an equal level, and your lost relationship with the Supreme Personality of Godhead is again established. Then your real life begins.

Taking up Kṛṣṇa consciousness means that we begin our real life and get free from the temporary life of changing from one body to another. So the Kṛṣṇa consciousness movement is a very important movement. Try to understand it. We have our magazine, *Back to Godhead*, and we have branches in many places in your country .

So we invite you to come. There is no expenditure. We simply request that you come and try to understand this movement. It is very scientific; it is not a bogus bluff. Try to understand with all your argument, reason, logic. We are prepared to answer your questions.

This movement is for your benefit; it is not an institution to make some profit. It is just meant to render service to the whole of humanity so that you may understand the science of God and be benefited. We are simply presenting Kṛṣṇa consciousness before you. Now it is up to you to accept it or not. Thank you very much.

Are there any questions?

Student: How does Kṛṣṇa consciousness relate to *advaita* philosophy?

Śrīla Prabhupāda: The basic principle of *advaita* philosophy is that the living being is one with God. That is a fact. We are nondifferent from God. For example, the president of your country is an American, and you are also an American. So there is no difference between you as far as being Americans is concerned. In that sense you are one. But at the same time, you are not the president. That you are an American does not mean you are on an equal level with the president. Is that not a fact?

Similarly, we are all qualitatively one with God. The word *qualitatively* means that whatever we have as spirit souls, God also has. There is no difference in quality. For example, suppose you take a drop of water from the vast Atlantic Ocean and you chemically analyze the ingredients. The composition of the drop of water is the same as the composition of the vast Atlantic Ocean. So qualitatively the drop of water is equal to the vast mass of water in the Atlantic Ocean. Similarly, you are a spirit soul, a spark of the supreme spirit soul, God. You have all the spiritual qualities that God has. But God is great, you are minute. He is infinite, you are infinitesimal. So you and God are qualitatively one but quantitatively different.

Those who are simply accepting the feature of being qualitatively one with God—they are called *advaita-vādīs.* They forget that quantitatively they cannot be equal to God. If the living entity is quantitatively equal to God, then why has he fallen into this miserable conditioned life of material existence? Because the living entity's constitutional position is infinitesimal, he is prone to be caught up by the influence of *māyā,* illusion. How could he be caught by *māyā* if he is also the Supreme? Then *māyā* would be greater than God. These things are to be considered.

So our philosophy, the Vedānta philosophy, is *acintya-bhedābheda-tattva,* inconceivable simultaneous oneness and difference between God and the living entity. We are qualitatively one with God, but quantitatively we are different. That is our philosophy, Vaiṣṇava philosophy. So *advaita-vāda* (oneness) and *dvaita-vāda* (difference) are both true. We are nondifferent from God in quality, but different in quantity. That is perfect philosophy.

Is that clear to you?

Student: Well, I heard someone give an analogy that we're just like rivers flowing into the sea. The sea is Brahman, the Absolute, and when we reach enlightenment we merge into Brahman and become one with the pure light and the spirit.

Śrīla Prabhupāda: But although water is always being poured into the sea, water is also being taken out. That is a fact. From the sea, water evaporates and forms a cloud, and from the cloud water again falls down into the sea as rain. Sea water is not in a fixed position.

So do not think that because you have once mixed with the sea water there is no chance of coming out again. You have to come out. But if you enter within the sea water and become one of the aquatics there, you don't have to come out. So our philosophy is not to mix with the water but to go deep into the water and become one of the aquatics there. Then we won't have to come out again.

The *Śrīmad-Bhāgavatam* [10.2.32] says,

ye 'nye 'ravindākṣa vimukta-māninas
tvayy asta-bhāvād aviśuddha-buddhayaḥ
āruhya kṛcchreṇa paraṁ padaṁ tataḥ
patanty adho 'nādṛta-yuṣmad-aṅghrayaḥ

This is a very nice verse. It says that although some people think they have become liberated by Brahman realization, their hearts are not yet purified, because they reject the service of Kṛṣṇa. Therefore, even after performing severe austerities and entering the Brahman effulgence, they must come back again to the material world. So if you don't want to come back again, then you have to enter deep into the "water" of the spiritual kingdom and remain as one of the servants of the Lord. This is the Vaiṣṇava philosophy.

We want to enter into the spiritual kingdom and live in our spiritual identity. We don't want to superficially mix with water and again evaporate, again come back. Those who believe in the philosophy of *advaita-vāda* generally give the example you have given, but any sane man can understand that mixing superficially with the water of Brahman is not perfection. Then you must come out again by evaporation. If you want to use that example, you have to also accept this conclusion. How can you say you are not coming back? It is a fact .

So if you don't want to come back again, go deep into the water and become one of the living entities under the shelter of the water. They have no problem; they do not come back. The big aquatics live peacefully within the water. They never come out into the rivers, because in the rivers there is no place to accommodate them. So if you want to live perpetually in the spiritual kingdom, you have to understand your identity as one of the servants of God. Then you'll be perfect.

Thank you very much.

The Human Machine

Like any machine, the human body has a purpose. Śrīla Prabhupāda explains what it is: "If in this life I practice chanting the Hare Kṛṣṇa mantra, *then gradually the core of my heart will be cleansed and everything will become manifest. My position, my duty, what is God—everything will become clear." (July 1975, Philadelphia)*

niśamya mriyamāṇasya mukhato hari-kīrtanam
bhartur nāma mahārāja pārṣadāḥ sahasāpatan

"My dear king, the order carriers of Viṣṇu, the Viṣṇudūtas, immediately arrived when they heard the holy name of their master from the mouth of the dying Ajāmila, who had certainly chanted without offense because he had chanted in complete anxiety" [*Śrīmad-Bhāgavatam* 6.1.30].

In your city the police are wandering in their car, and if somebody calls for the police, immediately they go to him. Similarly, the attendants of Lord Viṣṇu are wandering throughout the universe, searching out somebody who is chanting the holy name of the Lord. If you chant the holy name of the Lord, they are very much pleased, and they immediately come.

When Ajāmila called out "Nārāyaṇa!" he was simply calling his son, but the attendants of Hari took notice only of the chanting, that's all. They did not care to know whether or not Ajāmila meant Lord Nārāyaṇa. No. Because they heard their master's name, they immediately appeared. This is clear.

So, anyone who chants the holy name of the Lord is immediately taken care of by the attendants of the Supreme Lord. Especially if one chants at the time of death—that is when the account is figured up. If you practice chanting Hare Kṛṣṇa during your lifetime, naturally at the last moment of your life you will be inclined to chant Hare Kṛṣṇa. It is so nice.

If in this life I practice chanting the Hare Kṛṣṇa *mantra,* then gradually the core of my heart will be cleansed and everything will become manifest. My position, my duty, what is God—everything will become clear (*ceto-darpaṇa-mārjanam*). Now, because our hearts are filled up with so much rubbish, we cannot understand the science of God. But if you practice chanting the Hare Kṛṣṇa *mahā-mantra,* your heart will become cleansed and you will see things as they are.

And as soon as you are able to see things as they are, your material bondage is over. Now you are researching the bodily senses—finding out how they work—and doing so many things simply on the basis of the body. But as soon as your heart becomes cleansed, you will immediately understand, "I am not this body. So what is the use of studying cells and atoms, this and that? I am simply wasting my time."

Suppose I am driving a very nice car, but I am simply absorbed in the machine only. I have forgotten my destination, where I have to go, and I am busy studying the car. What is the use? You may be driving a good car, but you must know how to reach your destination. That is your main business. Knowing how the car works is secondary. Your main business is knowing how to utilize the car so you can reach your destination. That is intelligence.

So, we have fallen into this material condition, and we are occupying various forms. As long as we are in the bodily concept—thinking "I am this 'car'"—that is ignorance. What is wanted is to think, "I am not this body. I am spirit soul, and I have to utilize this body to go to my destination—the spiritual world—where I can meet the supreme spirit, God, and live in His association." Human life is meant for understanding what the Supreme Lord is, where He lives, what He does, and what our relationship with Him is. To seek to understand these things is called *brahma-jijñāsā,* "inquiry into the Absolute Truth." That is actual education.

We are given this machine of the body, but what is the use of simply studying the machine? The *śāstra* [scripture] says that since the machine will work until it is rotten, you shouldn't bother with the machine but should search out the Absolute Truth. But people are simply thinking, "Oh, now we have such a good machine." The dog also has a machine. The ant also has a machine, the elephant has a machine, the human being has a machine—every living entity has a bodily machine. But the *śāstra* says that this human machine should not be utilized like the animals'.

God has given us a human machine, and now we should use it to go to our destination. *Nṛ-deham ādyaṁ . . . plavaṁ su-kalpam.* This *nṛ-deha,* this human machine, is very carefully made—not by me but by nature. Nature is the agent of God. I wanted to do something, and so I required a particular type of machine. God ordered nature: "This living entity wants to do such and such, so give him an appropriate machine." And she did that.

So, *prakṛti,* or nature, gives us different types of machines. *Prakṛteḥ kriyamāṇāni guṇaiḥ karmāṇi sarvaśaḥ.* I am not the ultimate controller of the machine, nor have I made the machine. Rather, I have been given this machine as a gift to fulfill my desires. This is our position.

Now, the *śāstra* says, *nṛ-deham ādyaṁ su-labhaṁ su-durlabhaṁ plavaṁ su-kalpam.* This human body is a very good machine, and it is very rare. With great difficulty we have gotten this machine, because we had to come through so many other machines—the aquatics, the plants, the insects and trees, the serpents and reptiles, and then the birds and beasts. This has taken millions and millions of years. We have seen trees that are standing for more than five thousand years. If you get that kind of machine, you cannot move: you have to stand in one place. We had to go through this. Foolish people do not know.

Therefore this human machine is *su-durlabham,* "very difficult to attain." And it is also *su-kalpam,* "very nicely made." Those who are medical men know how nicely it is made—how the nerves are working, how the muscles are working, how the brain is working, how the intestines and heart and everything is working so nicely. It is a grand machine. Therefore it is *su-kalpam,* "very well constructed."

And what for? Suppose you have a nice, well-constructed boat. Then you can get into it and cross over a river or ocean. Similarly, in the human "boat" we can cross over this material ocean. Life after life we have been struggling in this material ocean, but now we have a suitable boat to cross it—this human body.

The human boat is especially advantageous because the breeze is very favorable. The breeze is the *śāstra,* or bona fide scripture. When you ply your boat, if the breeze is favorable for pushing on to your destination, that is another advantage. So, we have a good boat and a good breeze. And, *guru-karṇadhāram*—the guru is the good captain who can steer the boat. He is giving instructions: "Sail like this, turn quickly this way, now that way."

So, we have a great opportunity: the boat is very nice, the captain is very good, the breeze is very favorable. But if with all these advantageous facilities we do not cross over the sea of ignorance, of material existence, then we are committing suicide (*sa ātma-hā*). You have such a great opportunity, yet still you are remaining in this material world, repeatedly suffering birth, old age, disease, and death. Is that very good intelligence?

People are being misled. They are studying the human machine, that's all. Instead of taking advantage of the machine to cross over the material ocean, they are busy studying it. And they cannot even study it completely. I may claim, "This is my body," but if somebody asks me, "How many hairs do you have on your body?" I cannot say. How I am eating something, how it is being turned into some secretion, how the secretion is becoming blood and going to the heart, how the blood is being distributed throughout the arteries and veins—I do not know any of these things. I can simply theorize.

The human machine is not under your control. The machine is made by God, or by nature, God's agent. It is a very subtle machine. So if you are intelligent, you will ask, "What is the use of simply studying the machine? I have it, so let me utilize it for going to my destination." That is intelligence.

But no, people neglect to use the human machine for going to their destination, and instead they simply study it. And this is going on in the name of science. What is this nonsensical science? Simply busy in studying the machine?

This is the mistake: Although we should use our developed human consciousness for going back home, back to Godhead, we are not doing so. Why should we waste our human intelligence? Suppose you study the human machine throughout your whole life. What will you get? Can you adjust the machine so it will not be lost, so there will be no death? All you scientists who are studying the machine, have you found any means by which there will be no death? Where is that knowledge? Death will come. You may study the machine or not study the machine, but in due course of time death will come and take you.

You cannot cure even one disease. You are embarrassed by the cancer disease. So, find out how the cells are working and how they can be changed, and then there will be no more cancer. No, that you cannot do. You go on studying and simply waste your time.

The *śāstra* says, "Don't waste your valuable time in that way. Try to understand God. Use your intelligence for this purpose." It is also said, *tapo divyam . . . yena sattvaṁ śuddhyet.* You have to undergo austerities so that in the future you will not be subjected to this machine. That is your business—not to study the machine, but to become independent of the machine.

As long as you are in this material world, you are desiring in a certain way, nature is supplying you a certain type of machine, then you are busy trying to fulfill your desires, then the machine breaks, and then you accept another machine. This is going on. So your problem is to stop this repetition of birth, old age, disease, and death. Come to your spiritual life. That is your business. That is the instruction of the *śāstra*.

Everyone knows how to maintain the machine. The dog

knows how to maintain his machine. He eats according to the necessity of his doggish body. Similarly, we are maintaining our human body. That is natural. The supplies are already there. You cannot manufacture them. That is the Vedic instruction: *nityo nityānāṁ cetanaś cetanānām eko bahūnāṁ yo vidadhāti kāmān.* "There are millions and trillions of living entities, but there is one living entity—God—who is supplying the necessities of all the others."

We ordinary living entities have many millions of duplicates. Therefore the word *nityānām* is used, meaning "eternal living beings." The ordinary living beings, or *jīvas,* are innumerable. You cannot count them. But above these innumerable living entities is one prime living entity, God. He is also a living entity, as we are. In your Bible there is the statement that "Man is made in the image of God." So, God is a living entity, and this human form is made according to the form of the Lord. The human form is an imitation; God's form is real (*sac-cid-ānanda-vigraha*).

But you are thinking that God has no form. Why? Wherefrom did you get your form? You are praying daily, "O God, our father, give us our daily bread." So, you accept God as the supreme father. And if you have form, your father must have form. This is reasonable. Therefore how can you say God has no form? This is all foolishness.

Suppose a child is born after the death of his father. So, simply because he has not seen his father, that does not mean he should conclude, "My father had no form." This is not a good conclusion. His mother can tell him, "Yes, my child, your father had form." This is intelligence.

So, God is a living entity, but the difference between Him and all the other living entities is that they are all dependent on Him. That's all. God is great, we are small. He is just like a father who maintains all his children. We are all children, and the supreme father maintains us.

Now, one child may like to play with a motorcar toy, another with a doll, and so on. And the parents are supplying: "All right, you take this toy car, you take this doll." Similarly, we are playing like that—making plans to enjoy—and God is supplying all our necessities. But He doesn't want to do that. He says, "My dear child, you are grown up now; you have this human body. Don't play like this and waste your time. Get an education and know things as they are." That education is called *brahma-jijñāsā,* "inquiry into the Absolute Truth." As the *Vedānta-sūtra* says, "Now that you have the human form of life, try to understand God. That is your main business."

Unfortunately, we are misled by blind leaders. We have been engaged in studying the body, that's all. So here it is said, *niśamya mriyamāṇasya mukhato hari-kīrtanam.* God very much appreciates it when we use our tongue and mouth to chant His holy name. He very much appreciates that. Because the name of God is not different from God Himself, as soon as you chant Hare Kṛṣṇa you are in touch with Him.

In another place the *Bhāgavatam* says, *puṇya-śravaṇa-kīrtanaḥ. Śravaṇa* means "hearing," and *kīrtanaḥ* means "chanting." So, one who is chanting God's name and one who is hearing God's name—both are purified. Simply by chanting the name of God one can be delivered from birth and death. The example is given here—Ajāmila. He was addicted to so many sinful activities, and out of fear or because of good luck he chanted "Nārāyaṇa!" at the time of death. Immediately the attendants of Nārāyaṇa came to deliver him. This is the great benefit of chanting the holy name of the Lord.

Hare Kṛṣṇa. Thank you very much.

The Sense to Know God

Tasting and talking—two things we do many times a day—turn out to be the easiest and quickest means to God realization. We simply need to know what to taste and vibrate. Śrīla Prabhupāda explains in this lecture given in Hamburg, Germany, in 1969.

> *viṣṇu-śaktiḥ parā proktā kṣetra-jñākhyā tathā parā*
> *avidyā-karma-saṁjñānyā tṛtīyā śaktir iṣyate*

"Lord Viṣṇu's potency is summarized in three categories—namely, the spiritual potency, the living entities, and ignorance. The spiritual potency is full of knowledge; the living entities, although belonging to the spiritual potency, are subject to bewilderment; and the third energy, which is full of ignorance, is always visible in fruitive activities."

This verse from the *Viṣṇu Purāṇa* states that the energy of the Supreme Lord (*viṣṇu-śakti*) is originally spiritual but that it manifests in three ways. It is like the sunshine, the energy of the sun globe. The sunshine is one energy, but it manifests as illumination and heat. Similarly, God has one energy, which is spiritual and which sustains His spiritual abode. And that same energy is manifested in another spiritual form, the *kṣetra-jña*, or marginal energy, which comprises us living entities. Then, *avidyā-karma-saṁjñānyā tṛtīyā śaktir iṣyate:* "Besides these two forms of the Lord's energy there is a third form, known as *avidyā,* or ignorance, which is based on fruitive activities." One who is influenced by this energy has to experience the good and bad fruit of his labor. This is the material world. The material world is also an energy of Kṛṣṇa, or God, but here ignorance prevails. Therefore one has to work. In our original state we haven't got to work, but when we are in ignorance we have to work.

So, Kṛṣṇa actually has one energy, the spiritual energy. He is the whole spirit, and the energy emanating from Him is also spiritual. *Śakti-śaktimator abhedaḥ*. From the *Vedānta-sūtra* we learn that the energetic, Lord Kṛṣṇa, is nondifferent from His energy. Therefore the material energy is also nondifferent from Kṛṣṇa. In another place in the Vedic literatures it is said, *sarvaṁ khalv idaṁ brahma:* "Everything is Brahman, spirit." And in the *Bhagavad-gītā* [9.4] Kṛṣṇa says, *mayā tatam idaṁ sarvaṁ jagad avyakta-mūrtinā:* "I am expanded as this cosmic manifestation, My impersonal feature." *Mat-sthāni sarva-bhūtāni na cāhaṁ teṣv avasthitaḥ:* "Everything is resting on Me, or everything is an expansion of Myself, but personally I am not there."

This is *acintya-bhedābheda,* the philosophy of simultaneous oneness and difference of God and His energies. Inaugurated by Śrī Caitanya Mahāprabhu, although it is there in the aphorisms of the *Vedānta-sūtra,* this philosophy can satisfy the two classes of philosophers who study the Absolute Truth. One class says that God and the living entities are different, and the other philosophers, the monists, say God and the living entities are one. This *acintya-bhedābheda* says that God and the living entities are simultaneously one and different. They are one in quality, but different in quantity.

Again we can give the example of the sunshine and the sun globe—the energy and the energetic. In the sunshine there is heat and illumination, and in the sun globe there is also heat and illumination. But the degrees of light and heat are quite different. You can bear the heat of the sunshine, but if you went to the sun globe you could not bear the heat there; it would immediately burn everything to ashes. Similarly, Kṛṣṇa and the living entities are quantitatively very different.

Kṛṣṇa is infinite, while we are smaller than the atom. Therefore we cannot possibly know the Supreme Personality of Godhead by our ordinary sense perception. *Ataḥ śrī-kṛṣṇa-nāmādi na bhaved grāhyam indriyaiḥ:* "Kṛṣṇa isn't perceivable by our blunt material senses." The word *nāmādi* means "beginning with His name." With our material senses we cannot understand Kṛṣṇa's names, form, qualities, paraphernalia, or activities. It is not possible.

Then how are they to be understood? *Sevonmukhe hi jihvādau svayam eva sphuraty adaḥ:* "When we render transcendental loving service to the Lord with our senses, beginning with the tongue, the Lord gradually reveals Himself." Our first business is to engage the tongue in the service of the Lord. How? By chanting and glorifying His name, fame, qualities, form, paraphernalia, and pastimes. This is the business of the tongue. When the tongue is engaged in the service of the Lord, all the other senses will gradually become engaged.

The tongue is the most important sense within the body. Therefore it is recommended that if we want to control our senses we should first control the tongue. Śrīla Bhaktivinoda Ṭhākura has emphasized this. He describes our present conditioned state as *śarīra avidyā-jāl:* we are packed up in the network of this material body, and we are just like a fish caught within a net. And not only are we caught in this body; we are also changing this "net" life after life, through 8,400,000 species. In this way we stay caught in the network of ignorance. Then, *joḍendriya tāhe kāl:* our imprisonment within this network of ignorance is being continued on account of our desire for sense enjoyment. And out of all the senses, Bhaktivinoda Ṭhākura says, the tongue is the most dangerous. If we cannot control the tongue, then the tongue will oblige us to take different types of bodies, one after another. If a person is very much fond of satisfying his tongue by eating flesh and blood, then material nature will give him the facility to regularly taste fresh flesh and blood: he will get the body of a tiger or some other voracious meat-eating animal. And if one does not discriminate in his eating—if he eats all kinds of nonsense, everything and anything—then material nature will give him a hog's body, in which he will have to accept stool as his food. So much suffering is caused by the uncontrolled tongue.

Therefore, this human body is a great opportunity, because by engaging the tongue in the loving service of the Lord we can advance in Kṛṣṇa consciousness. We can achieve ultimate realization of God just by engaging the tongue in His service. In other bodies—the cat's body, the dog's body, the tiger's body—we cannot do this. So this human form of life is a great boon to the living entity, who is traveling through the cycle of birth and death, perpetually inhabiting different sorts of bodies. The human body is the opportunity for utilizing the tongue properly and getting out of the clutches of the material nature.

If we can keep our tongue always engaged in chanting the Hare Kṛṣṇa *mantra,* we will realize Kṛṣṇa, because the sound of Kṛṣṇa's name is not different from Kṛṣṇa Himself. Why? Because Kṛṣṇa is absolute. In the material world, everything is different from its designation. I myself am different from my name and from my body. But Kṛṣṇa is not like that: Kṛṣṇa and His name are the same, and Kṛṣṇa and His body are the same. The rascals cannot understand this. As Kṛṣṇa says in the *Bhagavad-gītā* [9.11], *avajānanti māṁ mūḍhā mānuṣīṁ tanum āśritam:* "Rascals and fools deride Me when I appear as a human being. They think I am an ordinary human being." *Paraṁ bhāvam ajānanto mama bhūta-maheśvaram:* "These rascals do not know what I am. They do not know My transcendental nature and My supreme influence over the entire creation."

Without understanding Kṛṣṇa, the fools consider Him an ordinary human being. The word *mūḍhā* in this verse from the *Bhagavad-gītā* means "rascal." Yet in spite of this warning, there are so many rascals passing as big scholars. When Kṛṣṇa orders "Surrender to Me," the rascals comment, "It is not to Kṛṣṇa but to the unborn spirit within Kṛṣṇa that we have to surrender." They do not know that Kṛṣṇa is not different from His body, that Kṛṣṇa is not different from His name, and that Kṛṣṇa is not different from His fame. Anything pertaining to Kṛṣṇa *is* Kṛṣṇa. These rascals are monists, philosophizing about "oneness," but as soon as they come to Kṛṣṇa they immediately try to separate Him from His body or from His name.

But the fact is that Kṛṣṇa's name and Kṛṣṇa are not different. Therefore, as soon as your tongue touches the holy name of Kṛṣṇa, you are associating with Kṛṣṇa. And if you constantly associate with Kṛṣṇa by chanting the Hare Kṛṣṇa *mantra*, just imagine how purified you will become simply by this chanting process.

Our tongue also wants very palatable dishes to taste. So Kṛṣṇa, being very kind, has given you hundreds and thousands of palatable dishes—remnants of foods eaten by Him. And if you simply make this determined vow—"I shall not allow my tongue to taste anything not offered to Kṛṣṇa and shall always engage my tongue in chanting Hare Kṛṣṇa"—then all perfection is in your grasp. All perfection. Two simple things: don't eat anything not offered to Kṛṣṇa, and always chant Hare Kṛṣṇa. That's all.

Variety is the mother of enjoyment, and *kṛṣṇa-prasādam* [food offered to Kṛṣṇa] can be prepared in so many nice varieties. How much enjoyment do you want with your tongue? You can have it simply by eating *kṛṣṇa-prasādam*. And the more your tongue becomes purified by tasting *kṛṣṇa-prasādam,* the more you'll be able to relish chanting the Hare Kṛṣṇa *mantra*. As Lord Caitanya says, *ānandāmbudhi-vardhanam:* "Chanting Hare Kṛṣṇa increases the ocean of transcendental bliss." We have no experience within this material world of an ocean increasing. If the oceans would have increased, then all the land would have been swallowed up many long, long years ago. But the ocean of transcendental bliss produced by chanting Hare Kṛṣṇa is always increasing.

The great authority Śrīla Rūpa Gosvāmī says, "What good is chanting Hare Kṛṣṇa with one tongue? If I had millions of tongues, then I could chant to my full satisfaction. And what good are these two ears? If I had millions of ears, I could hear Hare Kṛṣṇa sufficiently." He's aspiring to have millions of ears and trillions of tongues to relish the chanting of Hare Kṛṣṇa. This is an elevated stage, of course, when the chanting is so sweet and melodious that we want to have more ears and more tongues to relish it.

At present, however, we cannot know how relishable the

name of Kṛṣṇa is (*ataḥ śrī-kṛṣṇa-nāmādi na bhaved grāhyam indriyaiḥ*). With our present senses we can't understand the name, form, and qualities of Kṛṣṇa. Therefore if we try to immediately understand Kṛṣṇa by looking at His picture, we shall think, "Oh, Kṛṣṇa is simply a young boy embracing Rādhārāṇī and the other *gopīs*." Unless our senses are purified, we shall accept the dealings between Kṛṣṇa and Rādhārāṇī as ordinary dealings between a young boy and a young girl. Actually, this is not the fact. Their dealings are completely pure.

In the *Caitanya-caritāmṛta*, Śrīla Kṛṣṇadāsa Kavirāja Gosvāmī explains that there is a gulf of difference between the loving affairs of the *gopīs* with Kṛṣṇa and the ordinary, lustful dealings of human beings. He has compared the *gopīs'* love for Kṛṣṇa to gold, and our so-called love here to iron. As there is a great difference between gold and iron, there is a great difference between the loving affairs of the *gopīs* with Kṛṣṇa and the mundane, lusty affairs between men and women or boys and girls. Love and lust are never equal.

Therefore, to understand Kṛṣṇa as He is we have to purify our senses. And to do that we should carefully follow the principles of *sevonmukhe hi jihvādau:* first of all engage in chanting Hare Kṛṣṇa, Hare Kṛṣṇa, Kṛṣṇa Kṛṣṇa, Hare Hare/ Hare Rāma, Hare Rāma, Rāma Rāma, Hare Hare. Don't try to understand the loving affairs of Rādhā and Kṛṣṇa with your present senses, but simply chant Their holy names: Hare Kṛṣṇa. Then, when the dust on the mirror of your heart is cleansed away, you will understand everything.

Thank you very much.

From Folly to Defeat

Do modern achievements spell success in the eyes of the enlightened? Śrīla Prabhupāda gives his verdict: "The dog is thinking, 'I am this body,' and the cat is also thinking, 'I am this body.' So if a human being thinks like that, then he remains in ignorance. And if you remain in ignorance, whatever you believe to be to your credit is not an achievement: it is defeat. This is to be understood." (September 1973, Stockholm, Sweden)

parābhavas tāvad abodha-jāto
yāvan na jijñāsata ātma-tattvam
yāvat kriyās tāvad idaṁ mano vai
karmātmakaṁ yena śarīra-bandhaḥ

"As long as one does not inquire about the spiritual values of life, one is defeated and subjected to miseries arising from ignorance. Be it sinful or pious, *karma* (fruitive activity) has its reactions. If a person is engaged in any kind of *karma,* his mind is called *karmātmaka,* colored with fruitive activity. As long as the mind is impure, consciousness is unclear, and as long as one is absorbed in fruitive activity, one has to accept a material body" [*Śrīmad-Bhāgavatam* 5.5.5].

In the previous verse Ṛṣabhadeva has said that madly striving for sense gratification and doing all kinds of sinful activity are not good. Atheists may say, "Suppose we get a material body and it's a little miserable. What is wrong with that? It will be finished. Then there will be no more pains and pleasures." That is also the Buddhist theory: The body is a combination of matter producing pains and pleasures. So make this body zero; then there will be no more pains and pleasures.

So Ṛṣabhadeva answers this point: "No, although this body will be finished, you'll have to accept another body. And as long as you continue to accept one body after another, your miserable condition of material existence will continue."

In the beginning of his instructions Ṛṣabhadeva said that the human body is not to be misused simply for sense gratification like the dogs and hogs. So now he says, *parābhavas tāvad abodha-jāto yāvan na jijñāsata ātma-tattvam:* "These rascals do not know that for want of knowledge of the soul (*ātma-tattvam*), everything they are doing will be defeated." They are thinking, "Now, by scientific advancement we are able to go to the moon. This is our achievement." Of course, I do not know whether they can go—at least they are trying. But Ṛṣabhadeva says, "That is not your achievement. That is your defeat." Why? Because they are simply wasting their time.

Even if they go to the moon, they'll be driven away. What is the use of such an attempt? They cannot stay there. So this endeavor to go there by so-called scientific advancement is simply defeat. What have they achieved by these excursions? Nothing. No tangible achievement. But Russia and America have spent billions of dollars to go to the moon.

Even if they go there, they'll still have to die—they'll have to give up the body—and they do not know where they'll be placed after death. That is in nature's hands. No one can dictate, "After death I shall go to that planet or this planet." No. You are completely under nature's control.

Everyone is ambitious, but simply by becoming ambitious can one become a very rich man or a very respectable man? That is not possible. One must qualify himself. Similarly, to go and live on another planet one must be qualified. You have to act according to the higher laws. But they do not believe that there is higher authority, that there is judgment. They blindly think they can do whatever they like. That is not good. This is defeat (*parābhava*).

So as long as one is not inquisitive to understand what he is, he will be defeated in life. And this is the condition in today's so-called civilization: Nobody is interested to know his real identity. From Sanātana Gosvāmī we get the perfect example of how to inquire into one's identity. When he first approached Śrī Caitanya Mahāprabhu, he asked the Lord: '*ke āmi', 'kene āmāya jāre tāpa-traya.'* This is a very nice question: "Kindly tell me what I am and why I am subjected to the threefold miseries of material existence. I do not want all these miserable conditions of life, but I am forced to accept them. Therefore, what is my position? Why am I forced to accept them?"

This is called *ātma-tattva jijñāsa,* inquiry into one's real identity: "What am I?" Nobody knows what he is. Everyone thinks, "I'm this body." Therefore he's *abodha-jātaḥ:* from his very birth he's a fool. He does not know his identity. Someone's thinking, "I'm an American," someone's thinking, "I'm an Indian," someone's thinking, "I'm a Russian." All these identifications are doggish identifications.

The dog is thinking, "I am this body," and the cat is also thinking, "I am this body." So if a human being thinks like that, then he remains in ignorance. And if you remain in ignorance, whatever you believe to be to your credit is not an achievement: it is defeat. This is to be understood.

One should be inquisitive into who he is. Sanātana Gosvāmī has set the example. He went to Caitanya Mahāprabhu and said, "Sir, people say I am very learned, but actually I do not know what I am. Please instruct me on this topic." Ask any so-called scholar, doctor, Ph.D. if he knows what he is. Professor Kotovsky in Moscow said, "After the body is finished, everything is finished." He does not know what he is—an eternal soul. This is the position of everyone. Therefore, the so-called scholars, learned men, whatever they are doing, they're being defeated because they do not know their identity. Unless you know your identity, how can you work toward the goal of your life? If you are mistaken about your identity, then whatever you are doing, you will be defeated.

Then Ṛṣabhadeva says, *yāvat kriyās tāvad idaṁ mano vai karmātmakaṁ yena śarīra-bandhaḥ:* "As long as your mind is absorbed in fruitive activity, you have to accept one material body after another." Everyone has a different type of mentality. The word *karmātmakam* refers to the general mentality that "I shall work very nicely, I shall get money, and I shall enjoy life." Those who are followers of Vedic ritualistic ceremonies are trying to enjoy in the next life also—by *puṇya kārya,* or pious activities. But pious activities are also karmic or fruitive activities. Therefore, according to our philosophy, not only are we uninterested in impious activities, we are not even interested in pious activities. This is our position.

By pious activities you can take birth in a very aristocratic or rich family. You can become a very learned scholar. You can become beautiful. You American or Western people are supposed to be very learned, advanced in material science. You are also good-looking and richer than people in other countries. This is due to your past pious activities.

Suppose you have received these opportunities due to your past pious activities. Now, somebody else has taken birth in Greenland, where there is always snow and there are so many inconveniences. And someone else has taken birth somewhere in Africa where there are no facilities like those you have. From the spiritual point of view, all these situations are equivalent. In any birth, you have to enter within the womb of a mother to stay nine months in a packed-up condition. And nowadays they are killing the child within the womb. You may not even come out. Before you come out of your mother's womb you might be killed by your very mother or father. So whether you are in the womb of a very rich mother or a poor mother, a black mother or white mother, a learned mother or a foolish mother, the pains due to staying within the mother's womb are the same.

And as soon as you accept some material body, you'll have to suffer further bodily pains. Then, at the time of death, the same painful condition is there for everyone. So it doesn't matter whether one is rich or poor, the material condition will cause one to suffer.

So, if you continue to absorb your mind in fruitive activities, nature will continue to give you material bodies life after life so that you can try to fulfill your unfulfilled desires. This has been going on perpetually. Therefore a life devoid of inquiry into your real identity is *parābhava,* defeat.

Your real business is to know that you are not this body; you are spirit soul, part and parcel of God, Kṛṣṇa. Your real business is to become Kṛṣṇa conscious, fully, and go back home, back to Godhead, to finish this business of repetition of birth and death. But who will understand this? Therefore it is said: *kṛṣṇa ye bhaje se baḍa catura.* One who has understood the meaning of the Kṛṣṇa consciousness movement must be very intelligent. Without being intelligent, nobody can understand the basic principle of this movement.

The basic principle of this movement is to understand Kṛṣṇa. And if you understand Kṛṣṇa, then after giving up this body, you go to Kṛṣṇa. Devotional service—chanting Hare Kṛṣṇa, worshiping Kṛṣṇa in the temple, and so on—all these activities will help you understand Kṛṣṇa. Although it is very difficult to understand Kṛṣṇa, if you engage yourself in Kṛṣṇa's service as prescribed in the *śāstras* or by the spiritual master, then Kṛṣṇa will reveal to you what He is. And that is the perfection of your life. As soon as you understand Kṛṣṇa, you become fit to go back home, back to Godhead, and finish this business of repeated birth and death.

This is confirmed by Lord Ṛṣabhadeva in the next verse:

evaṁ manaḥ karma-vaśaṁ prayuṅkte
avidyayātmany upadhīyamāne
prītir na yāvan mayi vāsudeve
na mucyate deha-yogena tāvat

"When the living entity is covered by the mode of ignorance, he does not understand the individual living being and the supreme living being, and his mind is subjugated to fruitive activity. Therefore, until one has love for Lord Vāsudeva, who is none other than Myself, he is certainly not delivered from having to accept a material body again and again."

So everyone has the wrong conception of life. But one can be saved if he somehow or other becomes a devotee of Vāsudeva, Kṛṣṇa. Ṛṣabhadeva is an incarnation of Vāsudeva.

In this entanglement of birth and death, if someone comes in contact with a devotee and gets the seed of devotional service, that is the beginning of his rescue from the repetition of birth and death. We are giving opportunity to the people in general, opening centers in many parts of the world. Why? To give everyone a chance to become a devotee of Vāsudeva, Kṛṣṇa. Then they will be saved.

People are struggling, working hard for sense gratification—and suffering repeated birth and death. In this struggle for existence, if somehow or other one gets the seed of devotional service to Vāsudeva, then he's saved. Unless one becomes Kṛṣṇa conscious, his repetition of birth and death—contacting one body after another—will continue. This understanding is the basic principle of Kṛṣṇa consciousness.

Do not think that Kṛṣṇa consciousness is a kind of religious faith. It is a science—the science of how to get release from the repetition of birth and death. It is not a system of religion, as people ordinarily accept some type of religion. Somebody's a Hindu, somebody's a Muslim, somebody's a Christian. It is not like that. It is a science. We are teaching, "Somehow or other, enhance your love for God. Then you are saved." And how do we enhance that love of Godhead? By our activities: rising early in the morning, chanting Hare Kṛṣṇa, studying the Vedic scriptures, worshiping the Deity in the temple, observing festivals honoring the Lord. These activities in devotional service will save us from the repetition of birth and death. Otherwise, we are doomed. We'll have to continue this repetition of birth and death.

Caitanya Mahāprabhu teaches that we are wandering throughout the universe from one body to another, one planet to another, due to *avidyā,* ignorance. But if somebody comes in contact with this Kṛṣṇa consciousness movement and tries to understand Kṛṣṇa consciousness, he's fortunate, because he'll be saved from the repetition of birth and death.

Therefore Kṛṣṇa personally comes, and He says, *sarva-dharmān parityajya mām ekaṁ śaraṇaṁ vraja:* "Give up everything else and just surrender unto Me." It is not Kṛṣṇa's interest for you to surrender. If you don't surrender, Kṛṣṇa does not lose anything. He's omnipotent. He can create whatever He wants by His desire. He's not canvassing, "You become My devotee, and I shall be very rich." No. It is for *your* interest. If you become a devotee of Vāsudeva, Kṛṣṇa, then you are saved from the repetition of birth and death.

It is Kṛṣṇa's interest in this way: because we are part and parcel of Kṛṣṇa, we are His sons. The rich father does not like to see his son become a crazy fellow loitering in the street. But if his son does not come home, there is no loss for the father. And if the son comes back to the home of his rich father, it is in the son's interest.

So Kṛṣṇa is canvassing: "Surrender unto Me." Those who are fortunate will accept this offer of Kṛṣṇa's. And when we actually love Kṛṣṇa, that is called *prīti*. We love our beloved—our child or husband or wife—but that is not real love. That is a temporary sentiment. Actual love is possible only with Kṛṣṇa. Once you love Kṛṣṇa, that love cannot be broken at any time. Therefore, somehow or other we have to engage ourselves in loving Kṛṣṇa. That is the success of life.

Thank you very much.

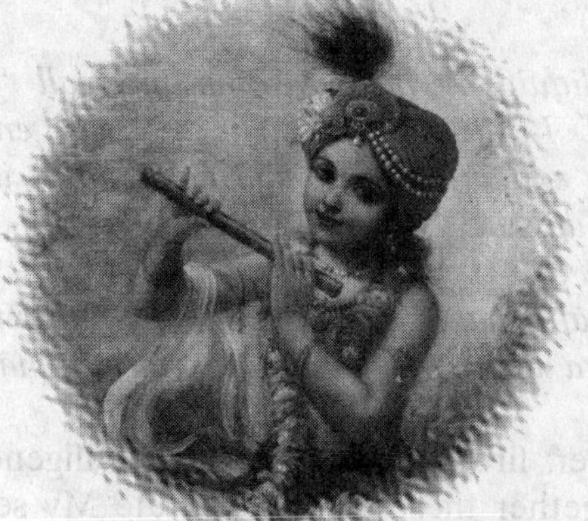

2.

Matter, Spirit, and the Controller of Both

From Matter to Spirit

Solids and liquids—what we commonly call "matter"—are just two of Lord Kṛṣṇa's eight material energies. Śrīla Prabhupāda explains how to spirtualize them in this lecture given in Vṛndāvana, India, in August 1974.

bhūmir āpo 'nalo vāyuḥ khaṁ mano buddhir eva ca
ahaṅkāra itīyaṁ me bhinnā prakṛtir aṣṭadhā

"Earth, water, fire, air, ether, mind, intelligence, and false ego—all together these eight constitute My separated material energies" [*Bhagavad-gītā* 7.4].

Here Lord Kṛṣṇa is explaining that He expands Himself by His material energies. Since these eight are His external energies, they are called *aparā,* "inferior." In the next verse Kṛṣṇa will explain that besides this inferior energy there is the superior energy, the living entities.

Because Kṛṣṇa is the supreme spirit soul, for Him there are no "superior" or "inferior" energies, but for us there are. For example, electricity can produce heat, and it can cool also. A refrigerator runs by electricity, and a heater also runs by electricity. So, we may say, "This is heat-producing electricity, and that is cold-producing electricity." But for the powerhouse there is no such distinction: It is all simply electricity. Similarly, for Kṛṣṇa there is no superior or inferior energy.

Now, Kṛṣṇa says that these eight energies are *His* energies. The materialistic scientists cannot understand that earth is Kṛṣṇa's energy, water is Kṛṣṇa's energy, and fire is Kṛṣṇa's energy. The scientists accept that these are different energies, but *whose* energies they are—that they do not know.

We should study Kṛṣṇa and Kṛṣṇa's energies very intelligently and analytically. For example, if we want to know how the vast ocean has come into existence, we can understand from the *Bhagavad-gītā* that this vast body of water has come from Kṛṣṇa's energy.

Now, try to understand how Kṛṣṇa's energy can produce such a large amount of water. First, consider that we produce perspiration from our body. That perspiration may be only one ounce of water, but it is produced from our body. How the water is coming out, I do not know. It is inconceivable. But it is coming out; that's a fact. Since I am a tiny living entity, I am always limited; therefore my energy is also limited. But Kṛṣṇa is unlimited. So He can produce unlimited perspiration from His body. We have to understand the ocean like that. Otherwise, it will not be possible for us to understand how such a vast amount of water has come into being.

All material elements are coming from a living entity, not from matter. For example, when the body is dead, the perspiration is not coming out, but as long as the body is living, the perspiration is there. Similarly, the source of all material elements is originally the supreme life—Kṛṣṇa—not matter.

One may ask why Kṛṣṇa calls the material elements—earth, water, fire, air, and so on—His "separated" energies. That He explains in a different verse [Bg. 9.4]: *mayā tatam idaṁ sarvaṁ jagad avyakta-mūrtinā.* The material energies are called "separated" because in this material world you cannot directly perceive the presence of the Supreme Personality of Godhead (*jagad avyakta-mūrtinā*). And then Kṛṣṇa says, *na cāhaṁ teṣv avasthitaḥ:* "I am not present there. Although the material world is made up of My energy, still I am not present there." This is the philosophy of *acintya-bhedābheda,* that Kṛṣṇa is simultaneously one with and different from His energies.

Now, each of these eight material elements is finer than the last one. Water is finer than earth. Earth does not move, but water can move. Therefore water is finer. But finer than water is fire, and finer than fire is air, and finer than air is ether, and finer than ether is mind, and finer than mind is intelligence, and finer than intelligence is *ahaṅkāra,* the ego, or identity. But even finer than the ego is the soul. The soul is of a very small magnitude, one ten-thousandth the tip of a hair (*keśāgra-śata-bhāgasya śatāṁśaḥ sādṛśātmakaḥ*).

Everything is explained in *Śrīmad Bhagavad-gītā*. If we accept it, we get full knowledge. In the first verse of this chapter [7.1] Kṛṣṇa says, *asaṁśayaṁ samagraṁ māṁ yathā jñāsyasi tac chṛṇu:* "Just hear Me. Then without any doubt you will understand Me in full."

Now, as we have mentioned, out of the eight material elements, the finest is *ahaṅkāra,* the ego. Ego cannot be abolished; it will always be there. But the ego has to be cleansed. Therefore the *bhakti-mārga,* the path of devotional service, is a cleansing process, a clearing process (*ceto-darpana-mārjanam*). The mind, the intelligence, the ego—everything remains, but they have to be cleansed. That is Caitanya Mahāprabhu's mission.

By chanting the Hare Kṛṣṇa *mantra* you'll be able to cleanse your misconception of life. Your misconception of life is to think, "I am matter—this material body." This is false ego. Actually, we are not matter. We are spirit soul. Therefore, pure ego is to know, *ahaṁ brahmāsmi:* "I am a spirit soul." That is the beginning of understanding. In the *Bhagavad-gītā* Kṛṣṇa describes this understanding as the *brahma-bhūta* platform—when one knows, "I am not this material body; I am a spirit soul."

So, gradually, by studying the teachings of the *Bhagavad-gītā* and practicing them in life, we shall very easily understand *ātma-tattva,* the science of the soul. That is the real business of human life. Unfortunately, we are not interested in understanding *ātma-tattva*. As Śukadeva Gosvāmī says to Mahārāja Parīkṣit in the *Śrīmad-Bhāgavatam* [2.1.2], *śrotavyādīni rājendra nṛṇāṁ santi sahasraśaḥ:* "My dear king, for ordinary men there are many subject matters for hearing." Who is that ordinary man? *Apaśyatām ātma-tattvaṁ:* one who has no interest in seeing what he is. Everyone is under the illusion that he is the body and that his bodily interests are his prime interests. But nobody is interested in the soul. Therefore people have so many books, so many newspapers, so many magazines they like to hear and read. But they are not interested in hearing the *Bhagavad-gītā* or

Śrīmad-Bhāgavatam, where *ātma-tattva,* the science of the soul, is described.

Why are they not interested? Śukadeva Gosvāmī says, *gṛheṣu gṛha-medhinām:* They are too absorbed in household affairs and are thinking, "This is life." They are thinking that they are happy within this material world. How? As Vidyāpati, a great Vaiṣṇava poet, has sung, *tātala saikate, vāri-bindu-sama suta-mita-ramaṇī-samāje. Suta* means "children," *mita* means "friends," and *ramaṇī* means "wife." So the happiness of material life is in society, friendship, and love. If we have many friends, and if there are a beautiful wife and nice children at home, then we think, "This is happiness; this is life." But that is not real life. Real life is to understand *ātma-tattva,* the science of the soul. Without understanding *ātma-tattva,* life is a failure.

We have created society, friendship, and love in this material world in order to become happy. Everyone wants to be happy because that is our natural inclination. We are part and parcel of Kṛṣṇa, and He is *ānandamayo 'bhyāsāt,* "by nature full of happiness." Kṛṣṇa is enjoying His life with Śrīmatī Rādhārāṇī and the other *gopīs* and the cowherd boys, and with His father and mother. All of that enjoyment is spiritual (*ānanda-cinmaya-rasa*).

Here in this material world we create an imitation: the same lovers, friends, parents, sons—but it is all false. In the desert an animal may see a vast mass of water, but it is only a mirage, and when the animal goes to drink the water, he dies. Similarly, in this material world we are trying to become happy by society, friendship, and love, but this is a will-o'-the-wisp, a false thing. Real life is in the society of Kṛṣṇa. Śrīla Bhaktivinoda Ṭhākura therefore says, *kṛṣṇera saṁsāra kara chaḍi anāche:* "If you enter into the society, friendship, and love of Kṛṣṇa, that is the perfection of life."

You will not find real happiness in earth, water, fire, air, and so on. They are Kṛṣṇa's separated energies. They are a reflection, a false representation—*chāyeva. Chāyeva* means "just like a shadow or reflection" For example, when you see your face in the mirror, it is not actually your face you are seeing. It is simply the reflection of your face. Similarly, this material world is just like a reflection of the real, spiritual world. Therefore it is known as Kṛṣṇa's separated energy.

Another example is a tape recording. If I speak into a tape recorder, when you play the tape my voice will come out. But that is not really my voice: it is a recording of my voice, my separated energy. With my energy I have spoken something—I have vibrated some sound—which is recorded on the tape. And when it is played back, it produces exactly the same sound, but still it is separated from me.

We should try to understand that this material world is Kṛṣṇa's separated energy. Real life is in the spiritual world. Therefore the *Śrīmad-Bhāgavatam* [1.1.1] says, *satyaṁ paraṁ dhīmahi:* "I meditate on the real truth, the Absolute Truth." Kṛṣṇa is the Absolute Truth, and in the *Bhagavad-gītā* He explains Himself. If we want to understand Kṛṣṇa, then instead of speculating about Him we should accept what He teaches about Himself. Then our knowledge will be perfect.

So, the fact is that this material world belongs to Kṛṣṇa—it is His separated energy—but we do not know how to use this energy for Kṛṣṇa. Kṛṣṇa's energy should be used for Kṛṣṇa's purposes. That is the Vaiṣṇava philosophy.

The Vaiṣṇava philosophy never says that this world is false. Why is it false? It is not false. The Māyāvādī [impersonalistic] philosopher says, *brahma satyaṁ jagan mithyā*: "The absolute is real; this world is false." Why is this world false? Take this temple, for example. If somebody says, "Yes, it is very nicely constructed, but it is all false," would we be happy? No. It is not false. What is this temple? It is Kṛṣṇa energy—a combination of earth, water, fire, air. This temple is made of bricks, but what is a brick? You take earth, mix it with water, and put it into the fire, and it becomes brick. And there is also air in this temple.

So this temple is Kṛṣṇa's energy. And it is not material, because it is being used for Kṛṣṇa. The Vaiṣṇava philosophy is that Kṛṣṇa's energy should be used for Kṛṣṇa's purpose, and when it is, it becomes spiritual. That is our philosophy.

The impersonalists, however, think that everything in this world is false and should be rejected. Śrīla Rūpa Gosvāmī describes this attitude as *phalgu-vairāgya,* false renunciation. In India there is a river named Phalgu. If you go there you'll see that there is no water on the surface of the river, but if you push your hand within the sand you'll touch water. So, *phalgu-vairāgya* means that a person renounces everything superficially but within his heart there is a desire to become God. He gives everything up, but he cannot give up this desire. This is the philosophy of the Māyāvādīs—to try to become one with God.

But the devotees do not try to become either one with God or separated from God. They are satisfied in whatever condition God puts them.

So, you have to understand that although this material energy is separated from Kṛṣṇa, it can be used for Kṛṣṇa. And when it is, it becomes spiritual. It is no longer material. It is material only when it is used in forgetfulness of Kṛṣṇa. When the *karmīs* [fruitive workers] construct a big, big skyscraper building, their purpose is to enjoy it themselves. They are using the same things we are using to build the temple—earth, water, fire, and air. They are mixing them together to make bricks and cement. But since the building is not being used for Kṛṣṇa, it is material. Only if the building is used for the purposes of Kṛṣṇa is it spiritual. This is proper renunciation, *yukta-vairāgya.*

The philosophy of Kṛṣṇa consciousness is that although the elements of this material world are separated form Kṛṣṇa, we can use them for Kṛṣṇa and thus spiritualize them. Again the same example: A tape recorder is material, but it can be used for Kṛṣṇa's purpose. That is how we are writing books—recording them on a tape recorder. This is *yukta-vairāgya,* proper renunciation. There is no need to give up this earth, water, fire, and air, as the Māyāvādī philosophers say. You can use them in Kṛṣṇa's service. After all, it is all Kṛṣṇa's energy.

Then, although this earth, water, fire, and air are Kṛṣṇa's separated energies, when we reconnect them by engaging them in the service of the Lord, they become spiritual. Another example: if you put an iron rod into a fire, the rod becomes warm, warmer, warmer, warmer. Then, when it is red-hot, it is no longer an iron rod: it is fire. Similarly, although everything in this material world is separated from Kṛṣṇa, if you engage the things of this world in the service of Kṛṣṇa, they are no longer material: they are spiritual. This is the philosophy of the Vaiṣṇavas.

If you always remember that everything, whatever you are using, is Kṛṣṇa's energy, you will be in Kṛṣṇa consciousness. We living entities are also Kṛṣṇa's energy. Kṛṣṇa will explain this in the next verse: *apareyaṁ itas tv anyāṁ prakṛtiṁ vidhi me parām.* "There is another, superior energy of Mine." What is that *parā-prakṛti,* that spiritual energy? *Jīva-bhūta,* the living entities. As matter is Kṛṣṇa's energy, the spirit soul is also Kṛṣṇa's energy. And there is another world, the spiritual world. That is also Kṛṣṇa's energy. Everything is Kṛṣṇa's energy.

So, when Kṛṣṇa's material energy is engaged in the service of Kṛṣṇa, it is converted into spiritual energy, exactly as the iron rod is converted into fire when held in the fire. We devotees of Kṛṣṇa are attempting to engage all of Kṛṣṇa's energies in His service and in this way change the material world into the spiritual world. That is the Kṛṣṇa consciousness movement.

Thank you very much.

The Potencies of the Omnipotent

What would you do if you were omnipotent? Only what you wanted to. And that's the position of Lord Kṛṣṇa. As Śrīla Prabhupāda explains, "Kṛṣṇa doesn't have to do anything. He is simply playing on His flute and enjoying with [His consort] Rādhārāṇī, that's all. He hasn't got to go to the office, to the factory. He is simply enjoying."(December 1973, Los Angeles)

yadā mukundo bhagavān imāṁ mahīṁ
jahau sva-tanvā śravaṇīya-sat-kathaḥ
tadāhar evāpratibuddha-cetasām
abhadra-hetuḥ kalir anvavartata

"When the Personality of Godhead, Lord Kṛṣṇa, left this earthly planet in His self-same form, from that very day Kali, who had already partially appeared, became fully manifest to create inauspicious conditions for those who are endowed with a poor fund of knowledge" (*Śrīmad-Bhāgavatam* 1.15.36).

When Lord Kṛṣṇa leaves this earth planet or appears here, He does so by His own potency. In the *Bhagavad-gītā* [4.6] Kṛṣṇa says, *sambhavāmy ātma-māyayā:* "I incarnate by My own potency." God has unlimited potencies (*parāsya śaktir vividhaiva śrūyate*), and learned scholars and saintly persons have accepted the idea of God's potencies. There are certain philosophers, however, who are of the opinion that God has no potency. But that is not a fact. From the Vedic literature we learn that God has unlimited potencies.

Now, how can we understand the Lord's potencies? One way is by the example of fire, which has two potencies, heat and light. A fire is in one place, but it expands its potencies of heat and light. That is within our experience; it is not very difficult to understand. Similarly, the sun also expands the potencies of heat and light. It is lying in one corner of the sky, but it expands its potencies throughout the universe. The sunshine is distributed all over the sky, all over the planetary system, and so are the sun's light and heat. The sun is 93 million miles away from us, but still we are feeling scorching heat—120 degrees, 135 degrees.

If even a material thing like the sun has so much potency, how much more potency must the Supreme Personality of Godhead have! His potency is *acintya,* inconceivable. That is the statement of the *Vedas:*

na tasya kāryaṁ karaṇaṁ ca vidyate
na tat-samaś cābhyadhikaś ca dṛśyate
parāsya śaktir vividhaiva śrūyate
svābhāvikī jñāna-bala-kriyā ca

"The Supreme Lord has no duty to perform, and no one is seen to be greater than or equal to Him. He has unlimited varieties of energy, which act automatically" [*Śvetāśvatara Upaniṣad* 6.8].

This is a description of the Absolute Truth, the Supreme Person. What kind of person? A person like you, working the whole day for money? No. *Na tasya kāryaṁ karaṇaṁ ca vidyate:* Kṛṣṇa doesn't have to do anything. He is simply playing on His flute and enjoying with Rādhārāṇī, that's all. He hasn't got to go to the office, to the factory. He is simply enjoying: *ānanda-mayo 'bhyāsāt.*

And we try to imitate Kṛṣṇa's enjoyment. Young boys and girls like to mix with each other and dance together. The same activities are there in Kṛṣṇa's pastimes. Kṛṣṇa is dancing with the *gopīs* [cowherd girls] in the forest, and you are dancing with your girlfriend in the nightclub. But your dancing will not give you satisfaction, because it is imitation. If you want real dancing, come to Kṛṣṇa. That is Kṛṣṇa consciousness.

We are trying to take the misled people from illusion to reality. The Māyāvādī [impersonalistic] philosophers say that there is no pleasure in dancing: "Make it zero; forget it." But we don't say that. We say that there is dancing in the original conception of the Absolute Truth. That is what the *Vedānta-sūtra* says: *janmādy asya yataḥ*. "The Absolute Truth is that from which everything has come." Whatever you are experiencing—wherefrom has it come? It has come from the Absolute. That is the meaning of "Absolute." But because here in the relative world dancing is pervertedly reflected and is not reality, you are confused, baffled.

In Paris there is a club for old men, all about to die. They come to the club and pay a fifty-dollar entrance fee so they can enjoy young girls and wine. They cannot actually enjoy, yet still they come. As it is said, *jarāgate kiṁ yuvatī nārī:* "When one is an old man, what is the use of mixing with young girls?" Still, the old men like to mix with young girls, although they do not really enjoy. Therefore they are unsatisfied, frustrated. This is the position of those who are trying to imitate Kṛṣṇa, whose powers are far beyond our imagination.

Kṛṣṇa is so great that He is simultaneously and inconceivably present in all places. He explains this in the *Bhagavad-gītā* [9.4]:

mayā tatam idaṁ sarvaṁ jagad avyakta-mūrtinā
mat-sthāni sarva-bhūtāni na cāhaṁ teṣv avasthitaḥ

"By My impersonal feature I am spread everywhere. Everything is resting on Me, but I am not in everything." It is a fact that everything is resting on Kṛṣṇa, just as all the planets are resting on the sunshine. It is a scientific fact that the planets are being maintained by the heat and light of the sun.

Now, what do we mean that "everything is resting on Kṛṣṇa"? Take this earth planet, for example. Everything on this planet—the trees, the rivers, the mountains, the cities, the cars—all of that is one unit, the earth planet. And there are millions and trillions of planets. How are they existing? They are existing on the sunshine. And wherefrom does the sunshine come? The sunshine comes from the sun, which comes from God. Therefore, indirectly everything depends on Kṛṣṇa's potency. As he says, *mat-sthāni sarva-bhūtāni:* "Everything is resting on My potency." *Na cāhaṁ teṣv avasthitaḥ:* "But personally I am not within everything." This is *acintya-bhedābheda-tattva:* The Lord is simultaneously one with and different from everything. This is our philosophy.

So, our point is that Kṛṣṇa, although situated in the spiritual world, works through His potencies, just as a rich man sits in his parlor and runs his business through his subordinates. He hasn't got to personally go to the office. We have seen Mr. Birla [a wealthy Indian gentleman] sitting in his home and running his businesses through his "potencies"—his secretaries, clerks, and so on. They are doing all the work; he hasn't got to work.

Similarly, because Kṛṣṇa is the Supreme Person, He hasn't got to work personally. He is always engaged in playing His flute and dancing with the *gopīs.* That's all. *Ānanda-mayo 'bhyāsāt:* He is simply enjoying.

So, Kṛṣṇa's potencies are working in both the spiritual and material worlds. How? I have already given the example of the sun. The sun is in the sky, and the sunshine is working. By the energy of the sunshine the leaves are coming out on the trees, and when there is no sunshine they are dropping. Everything depends on the energy of the sun. Similarly, everything depends on the energies emanating from Kṛṣṇa. As explained in the Vedic literature:

eka-deśa-sthitasyāgner jyotsnā vistāriṇī yathā
parasya brahmaṇaḥ śaktis tathedam akhilaṁ jagat

"Just as a fire situated in one corner of a room fills the whole room with heat and light, so the Absolute Truth, Kṛṣṇa, though situated in His own abode, pervades this entire universe with His potencies." Whatever you see in this cosmic manifestation is simply a demonstration of the potencies of the Lord.

So, we take our birth and accept our death, but not independently. We are under the control of the Lord's material potency. The Lord has many potencies, which have been divided into three categories. One is called the internal potency, one is called the external potency, and one is called the marginal potency. The external potency is this material world—so many universes, so many planets, stars, and so on. These are all manifestations of Kṛṣṇa's external potency. And then there is the internal potency, the spiritual world. That we cannot see; it is not within our experience. But we get information about the spiritual world from the *Bhagavad-gītā* [8.20]: *paras tasmāt tu bhāvo 'nyo 'vyakto 'vyaktāt sanātanaḥ.* "Beyond this material nature is another nature, which is eternal." This material nature is not eternal. Take your body, for example. It is not eternal. Similarly, this gigantic "body" of the universe is also not eternal. It has a date of creation and a date of dissolution. But the spiritual nature is eternal—it is never created or annihilated.

Now, we are the Lord's marginal potency. For example, when we walk on the shore of the Pacific Ocean, some days we find that the water is covering part of the beach, and some days we see it is open. There is no water on that part. So, that part which is sometimes covered and sometimes open is called "marginal." Similarly, as Kṛṣṇa's marginal potency, we are sometimes influenced by the material nature and sometimes by the spiritual nature.

Actually, we belong to the spiritual nature, but because we are minute spirit souls we have come in contact with this material nature somehow or other. This is an incompatible position for us, and so we cannot make a permanent adjustment here. Therefore we are getting one type of body and enjoying or suffering, and then another type of body, than another, and so on.

But if we like, since we are of the spiritual nature we can transfer ourselves to the spiritual world and remain there eternally. The eternal nature of the soul is described in the *Bhagavad-gītā* [2.20]: *na jāyate mriyate vā kadācit.* "The soul never takes birth or dies at any time." In other words, the soul is everlasting, eternal. Then what is death? Death is the annihilation of the material body, not of the soul. Therefore it is said here, *na hanyate hanyamāne śarīre:* "The soul is not dead after the annihilation of the body."

So, the conclusion is that because we are marginal—situated between the spiritual nature and the material nature—we have a tendency to come under the control of Kṛṣṇa's external, material energy and identify ourselves with this temporary, material body. Actually we are spiritual; our real nature is eternal. We never take birth and never die. But on account of our contact with the material nature, we are getting material bodies, which are always changing. Thus we have accepted birth and death as natural. But that is not our real nature.

At the present moment we are under the material nature, but if we try we can get out of this covering of material nature and come to the spiritual nature. That is Kṛṣṇa consciousness—to leave that marginal position and come onto the "land" so that there will be no disturbance from the "water." If you remain in the marginal position, sometimes you will be covered by water and sometimes you will be dry. But if you come a little forward to the land side, the ocean has no power to touch you.

Now, Kṛṣṇa is not like us. The present verse of the *Bhāgavatam* says that Kṛṣṇa left this world, but that does not mean He left this world as we leave it. Our leaving this world means that we leave this material body and accept another material body. Now we may have an American body, and in our next life we may be in a Russian body. An American who is fighting against the Russians in this life may get a Russian body in his next life. (This is the law of nature: *sadā tad-bhāva-bhāvitaḥ.* "Whatever one thinks of at the time of death determines his next life.") And then in his Russian body he will fight with the Americans, and in his next life he will again become an American. This is going on: *bhutvā bhutvā pralīyate.* Sometimes Russian, sometimes American, go on fighting, that's all. This is called *māyā,* illusion.

Everyone in this material world is under this illusion. The living entities are loitering in this material nature, sometimes in this body, sometimes in that body, sometimes this way, sometimes that way. Simply loitering. No one knows where to find shelter, where to find permanent life, permanent peace, permanent happiness. They are simply changing forms of government: electing one rascal, rejecting him, electing another rascal, and rejecting him. Because the candidates are all rascals, the people have no alternative but to elect a rascal. They are thinking, "By electing this rascal, we shall be happy." *Andhā yathāndhair upanīyamānāḥ:* The people are blind, and they are accepting leaders who are also blind. What will be the profit? If you are blind and you are led by another blind man, what will be the profit? Both of you will fall down into a ditch.

Therefore, if you want real happiness, you must accept the leadership of a man who has eyes to see. And whose eyes are open? The guru's. That is explained in the Vedic literature:

oṁ ajñāna-timirāndhasya jñānāñjana-śalākayā
cakṣur unmīlitaṁ yena tasmai śrī-gurave namaḥ

Everyone is blind, in the darkness of ignorance. So it is the guru's business to open their eyes, to help them see things as they are. That is the guru's business.

How can darkness be removed? By light. At night we cannot see. Everything is dark because the sun is not in the sky. But in the morning, as soon as the sun rises, we can see everything. Now, because we are in the darkness of ignorance, we cannot see things properly. The spirit soul exists and God exists, but now we cannot see them. We have to get the light of transcendental knowledge to see things as they are. That is wanted.

The Vedic literature therefore advises, *tamasi mā jyotir gama:* "Don't keep yourself in darkness; go to the light." This is possible in human life. In animal life you kept yourself in darkness because there was no possibility of coming to the light. If I invite all the dogs and cats in Los Angeles to come here and hear about the *Bhagavad-gītā,* they will not come, because they are animals. But if I appeal to the human beings, some may be interested. They should all be interested, but the times are so bad that almost nobody is interested. Still, a few people may be interested, but not the cats and dogs.

In the human form of life there is a necessity of coming to the light and making a solution to the problems of life. Therefore Kṛṣṇa appears in this world. He states in the *Bhagavad-gītā* [4.6], *prakṛtiṁ svām adhiṣṭhāya sambhavāmy ātma-māyayā:* "I appear in My transcendental form by My own energy." We are under the control of the material nature, but Kṛṣṇa is not under this control. That is to be understood. Therefore the present verse of the *Bhāgavatam* says, *jahau sva-tanvā. Sva* means "own," and *tanu* means "body." In other words, Kṛṣṇa left this world in His own transcendental body.

So, when Kṛṣṇa appears in this world or leaves it, He does so in His own transcendental body. For us there is a distinction between the soul and the body. I am a spiritual soul, but my body is material. This distinction is there because we are conditioned by the material body. But Kṛṣṇa is not conditioned by a material body. Therefore here it says *mahīṁ jahau sva-tanvā:* "He left in His own, original, spiritual body."

One so-called scholar who does not know Kṛṣṇa has written a commentary on the *Bhagavad-gītā* in which he tries to make a distinction between Kṛṣṇa's soul and His body. Kṛṣṇa says [Bg. 9.34], *man-manā bhava mad-bhakto mad-yājī māṁ namaskuru:* "Just think of Me, become My devotee, offer your obeisances unto Me, and worship Me." But this rascal commentator says it is not to the person Kṛṣṇa that we should offer obeisances but to the soul within Kṛṣṇa. Just see how ignorant he is! He does not know that for Kṛṣṇa there is no such division between His self, or soul, and His body. This fool is rascal number one, and yet he has written a commentary on the *Bhagavad-gītā* and is accepted as a scholar. And this nonsense is going on all over the world.

Therefore Kṛṣṇa says, *avajānanti māṁ mūḍhā mānuṣīṁ tanum āśritam:* "The rascals [*mūḍhās*] think that because I appear in a human form I am an ordinary human being." And then, *paraṁ bhāvam ajānanto:* "They do not know My great potency." Still, these rascals go on explaining the *Bhagavad-gītā*.

So, while for us there is a distinction between the body and the soul, for Kṛṣṇa there is no such distinction. Also, there is no distinction between Kṛṣṇa Himself and His Deity form made of stone. Why? Because the stone is Kṛṣṇa's energy. Earth, water, fire, air—everything is Kṛṣṇa's energy. That we have already explained. Therefore He can appear in any form, from anywhere, from anything. That is Kṛṣṇa's potency. So, you have to understand what Kṛṣṇa is. And as soon as you understand Kṛṣṇa in truth, you become liberated: *janma karma ca me divyam evaṁ yo vetti tattvataḥ/ tyaktvā dehaṁ punar janma naiti mām eti so 'rjuna.*

Here the *Bhāgavatam* says *mahīṁ jahau sva-tanvā:* "Kṛṣṇa left this world in His own, original body." Still, Kṛṣṇa *seemed* to leave His body just to befool the rascals. The rascals think Kṛṣṇa is like us, and therefore, to bewilder them, Kṛṣṇa left an illusory body so that they may go on thinking like that. But actually, here is the secret: *mahīṁ jahau sva-tanvā.* "Kṛṣṇa left this world in His original body."

Now, here it also says, *śravaṇīya-sat-kathaḥ:* "Talks about Kṛṣṇa are transcendental." If His body were like ours—if He had a material body—then what would be the use of hearing about His activities? We are interested in the words of Kṛṣṇa in the *Bhagavad-gītā,* but if Kṛṣṇa were like us, why should we be interested? Actually, by hearing about Kṛṣṇa or from Kṛṣṇa you become liberated. So He cannot possible be an ordinary human being like us. Only the less intelligent class of men (*apratibuddha-cetasām*) think in this way.

The *Bhāgavatam* verse ends with the words *kalir anvavartata:* "Because Kṛṣṇa passed away, Kali [the personification of the present Age of Quarrel] got the opportunity to enter." That is to some extent a fact. But if Kṛṣṇa is everywhere, how can He go away? Kṛṣṇa can remain with you eternally. And if by becoming Kṛṣṇa conscious you keep yourself with Kṛṣṇa, where is the chance of Kali entering? So keep yourself always in Kṛṣṇa consciousness. Kali will not be able to touch you.

Hare Kṛṣṇa. Thank you very much.

The Fall of the Soul

Here Śrīla Prabhupāda explains that we belong in the spiritual world with Kṛṣṇa but that we have created our fearful condition in the material world just as a person creates a fearful situation in a dream. Responding to our desire, Kṛṣṇa has given us a chance to forget Him. (April 1972, Tokyo)

śrī-śuka uvāca
ātma-māyām ṛte rājan parasyānubhavātmanaḥ
na ghaṭetārtha-sambandhaḥ svapna-draṣṭur ivāñjasā

"Śrī Śukadeva Gosvāmī said: 'O King, unless one is influenced by the bewildering energy of the Supreme Personality of Godhead, there is no meaning to the relationship of the pure soul in pure consciousness with the material body. That relationship is just like a dreamer's seeing his own body working'" [*Śrīmad-Bhāgavatam* 2.9.1].

Many people inquire, "How did the living entity, who was with Kṛṣṇa, fall into the material world?" That question is answered here. The fallen living entity's condition is due to the influence of the Lord's material energy. Actually, he has not fallen. An example is given: The moon appears to be moving when clouds pass in front of it. Actually, the moon is not moving. Similarly, the living entity, because he is a spiritual spark of the Supreme, has not fallen. But he is thinking, "I am fallen. I am material. I am this body."

The body has no connection with the soul. We can experience this. The body is changing, dying, but I am the same. The idea that we have a connection with the body is due to the influence of the illusory energy of Kṛṣṇa. That illusory energy develops when we forget Kṛṣṇa.

In other words, our illusory identification with the body is simply due to our forgetfulness of the Lord. We wanted to forget; we wanted to give up Kṛṣṇa and enjoy the material world. Therefore Kṛṣṇa is giving us the chance. For example, when you play a part in a drama, if you feel, "I am the king," then you can act very nicely. But if you feel, "I am Karandhara,"* then you cannot play a king so nicely. The feelings must be there. If you are playing the part of a king, you must believe you are the king and have his courage. You have to forget that you are Karandhara. Then you can play the part very nicely, and the audience will appreciate. But if you think "I am Karandhara playing the part of the king," then you cannot play the part convincingly.

So because we wanted to play the part of Kṛṣṇa, the supreme enjoyer, Kṛṣṇa is giving us the chance—"Yes, feel like Me." The feeling that "I am the master, I am the king, I am Kṛṣṇa, I am God" is created by Kṛṣṇa: "All right, since you want to play the part of a king, I shall train you in such a way."

The director of a play tries to create the feelings within you for the part you are playing. In my youth I played the part of Advaita Ācārya in a drama about Lord Caitanya. Our director, Amritlal Bose, repeatedly said to me, "Feel like Advaita Ācārya." So when I performed my part under his direction, all the people in the audience were crying. The play was artificial, but the effect on the audience was so nice.

Similarly, we have nothing to do with the material world, but we have been trained by the illusory energy to think, "I am an Indian," "I am an American," "I am an intellecutal," "I am a laborer" "I am this," "I am that," "I have to do this," "I have so many duties." These are all illusions. We have nothing to do with all this nonsense, but still we are taking it very seriously: "I have to do like that. I am this. I am that."

That is explained here: *ātma-māyām ṛte rājan parasyānubhavātmanaḥ.* "Unless one is influenced by the bewildering energy of the Supreme Personality of Godhead, there is no meaning to the relationship of the pure soul in pure consciousness with the material body." While dreaming a man may cry out, "Oh, there is a tiger, a tiger! Save me!" An awake man observing may say, "Where is the tiger? Why are

*A disciple in the audience.

you shouting?" But the dreaming man is actually feeling that a tiger has attacked him.

Therefore this verse gives the example of a dream: *na ghaṭetārtha-sambandhaḥ svapna-draṣṭur ivāñjasā*. There cannot be any meaning of the relationship of the soul and the body except that it is like a dreaming man creating an imaginary situation. He is dreaming that there is a tiger, and he is creating a fearful situation. Actually there is nothing to fear—there is no tiger. The situation is created by a dream.

Similarly, we have created the material world and material activity. People are running around—"Oh, I am the manager. I am the factory owner. I am this, I am that. We know his politics. We have to defeat our competitors." All these things are created just as a man creates a situation in a dream—*svapna-draṣṭur ivāñjasā*.

So when someone asks, "When did we come into contact with the material nature?" the answer is that we have not come into contact. By the influence of the external energy we *think* we are in contact. Actually we are not fallen. We cannot be fallen. We have simply created a situation in which we think we are fallen. Actually, Kṛṣṇa has given us that situation. Because we wanted to imitate Him, Kṛṣṇa has given us an opportunity: "All right, you want to imitate Me? You want to be an imitation king on the stage? So, feel like this. Play like this. Do like this. People will applaud—'Oh, what a very nice king.'"

So everyone in the material world is playing some part. "I want to be prime minister." "I want to be a very big business magnate." "I want to be a leader." "I want to be a philosopher." "I want to be a scientist." They are trying to play all these parts, and Kṛṣṇa is giving the opportunity—"All right."

But these things are all nonsense. Simply dreaming. When you dream, the next moment the dream is gone, and everything in the dream is finished. No more tiger, no more jungle. Similarly, as long as the body continues one may think, "I am a responsible leader; I am this; I am that," but as soon as the body is finished, these ideas are gone.

Kṛṣṇa says, *mṛtyuḥ sarva-haraś cāham:* "As death, I take everything away." Just think of your past life. Suppose you were a king or something like that. From the *Bhṛgu-saṁhitā* it was ascertained that I was a big physician in my last life, with a spotless character, no sins. I don't know. It may be. But I have no remembrance that I was a physician. So what do we know? I might have been a very big influential physician with a good practice, but where is it all now? All gone.

So our contact with matter is just like a dream. We are not fallen. Therefore, at any moment we can revive our Kṛṣṇa consciousness. We become liberated as soon as we understand, "I have nothing to do with matter. I am simply Kṛṣṇa's eternal servant." Sometimes when a fearful dream becomes intolerable, we break the dream. Similarly, we can break the material connection at any moment as soon as we wake up to Kṛṣṇa consciousness. "Oh, Kṛṣṇa is my eternal master. I am His servant." That's all. That is the way.

Thank you very much.

Purify Your Existence

In this talk given on the anniversary of the appearance of Śrīla Bhaktivinoda Ṭhākura, a pioneer of the Kṛṣṇa consciousness movement in the modern era, Śrīla Prabhupāda informs us, "To turn your home into Vaikuṇṭha, the spiritual world, is not difficult. You simply have to adopt the right method. Lord Kṛṣṇa provides everything we need to bring the spiritual world into our lives." (September 1973, Mumbai, India)

Five hundred years ago Lord Caitanya Mahāprabhu, Lord Kṛṣṇa Himself in the role of His own devotee, started the *saṅkīrtana* movement, or the movement for spreading the congregational chanting of the holy names of God. Bhaktivinoda Ṭhākura was the father of the *saṅkīrtana* movement within the last two hundred years. He was a householder and responsible government officer—a magistrate. And he was a great devotee and a great *ācārya,* or prominent spiritual master, in the disciplic succession of Caitanya Mahāprabhu.

Bhaktivinoda Ṭhākura wrote many devotional songs. In one song he has written, *ye-dina gṛhe, bhajana dekhi, gṛhete goloka bhāya:* "One day while performing devotional practices, I saw my house transformed into Goloka Vṛndāvana, the spiritual world."

As Kṛṣṇa is not material, so His home, Goloka Vṛndāvana, is not material. And although Kṛṣṇa stays in His abode, Goloka Vṛndāvana, He is also present everywhere. That is Kṛṣṇa's omnipotence. The *Brahma-saṁhitā* states,

eko 'py asau racayituṁ jagad-aṇḍa-koṭiṁ
yac-chaktir asti jagad-aṇḍa-cayā yad-antaḥ
aṇḍāntara-stha-paramāṇu-cayāntara-sthaṁ
govindam ādi-puruṣaṁ tam ahaṁ bhajāmi

Kṛṣṇa, Govinda, is everywhere by one of His plenary portions, known as Paramātmā, or Supersoul. He is situated in every universe and within everyone's heart. Not only is He within the heart of everyone, but He is within the atom.

Similarly, Kṛṣṇa's place, Goloka Vṛndāvana, is also spread everywhere. How? By the presence of Kṛṣṇa's devotees. Kṛṣṇa says,

nāhaṁ tiṣṭhāmi vaikuṇṭhe yogināṁ hṛdayeṣu vā
yatra gāyanti mad-bhaktāḥ tatra tiṣṭhāmi nārada

"I do not stay in Vaikuṇṭha-loka, the spiritual world, or within the hearts of the yogis. I stay where My devotees chant My glories" [*Padma Purāna*].

That is Kṛṣṇa's omnipotence. We pray to God the omnipotent, the omniscient, the omnipresent. God can be present everywhere simultaneously.

There is no difference between God and His place. Therefore Caitanya Mahāprabhu recommends, *ārādhyo bhagavān vrajeśa-tanayas tad-dhāma vṛndāvanam*. As Kṛṣṇa is worshipable, His place is also worshipable. Similarly, as He is all-pervading, His place is also all-pervading.

How can any place be changed into Vaikuṇṭha, or Goloka Vṛndāvana? By the chanting of the holy name of the Lord. Devotees are so powerful that by chanting the holy name of God they make the all-powerful Supreme Lord descend, along with His personal abode. Therefore Bhaktivinoda Ṭhākura sings, "One day while performing devotional practices I saw my house transformed into Goloka Vṛndāvana."

We also can change our homes into Vaikuṇṭha. That is not difficult: we simply have to follow the authorized process of Kṛṣṇa consciousness. How to do this is explained by Bhaktivinoda Ṭhākura: *kṛṣṇera saṁsāra kara chāḍi anācāra*. "Giving up all sinful activities, carry on your worldly duties only in relation to Lord Kṛṣṇa." *Anācāra* means "sinful activities." You cannot associate with God if you are sinful. In the *Bhagavad-gītā* Kṛṣṇa says, *yeṣāṁ tv anta-gataṁ pāpaṁ . . . bhajante māṁ dṛḍha-vratāḥ:* "Only one who is completely free from sinful life can worship Me with firm determination."

In our Kṛṣṇa consciousness movement we do not recommend that you give up your occupation, give up your wife and children, and become a *sannyāsī,* a renunciant. No, that is not our movement. Among us are not only *sannyāsīs* but also *brahmacārīs* [celibate students], *gṛhasthas* [married people], and *vānaprasthas* [retired people]. Everyone is welcome. Everyone can worship Kṛṣṇa. There is no rule that only a certain class—*brāhmaṇas* or *sannyāsīs* or *brahmacārīs* or Hindus—can take part. No. Kṛṣṇa is open to everyone. *Māṁ hi pārtha vyapāśritya ye 'pi syuḥ pāpa-yonayaḥ.* Kṛṣṇa is open even for a person born in a lower-grade family. One simply has to adopt the means to approach Him—namely, giving up sense enjoyment and practicing the purifying process of Kṛṣṇa consciousness.

Many devotional songs give this same instruction. Narottama Dāsa Ṭhākura has sung, *viṣaya chāḍiyā kabe, śuddha habe mana, kabe hāma heraba, śrī-vṛndāvana:* "When I am free from sense enjoyment and my mind is clear, I will be able to understand Vṛndāvana." *Viṣaya* means "sense enjoyment." One has to give up sense enjoyment to become purified.

To give up sense enjoyment does not mean, for example, that we cannot eat. There is no prohibition against eating, but you cannot eat anything until it is first offered to Kṛṣṇa. Our life in Kṛṣṇa consciousness means to be always the servant of Kṛṣṇa. As the servant eats remnants of food left by the master, we servants of Kṛṣṇa eat remnants of food left by Kṛṣṇa. That food is called *prasādam,* or the Lord's mercy.

We have to lead our life in such a way that we give up *anācāra,* forbidden things, sinful things. There are four main sinful activities. These are illicit sex, unnecessary animal-killing, intoxication, and gambling. We have to give up these four principles of sin. Then our life becomes pure.

If we give up these four principles and chant the Hare Kṛṣṇa *mantra,* we become pure. You can see the examples in members of the Kṛṣṇa consciousness movement. Many of those who have wholeheartedly accepted Kṛṣṇa consciousness were accustomed to all these sinful practices. That was their daily affair. But they have given these things up. Now anyone can see how saintly they are. One has to accept the principles of purification. Then one's life becomes perfect.

People do not know what the perfection of life is. They think that material advancement is perfection. No, that is not the perfection of life, because even if you make a nice material arrangement you cannot enjoy it for long. At any time you may be kicked out. So where is your perfection?

Suppose you have a nice apartment, a good bank balance, and a nice wife and children. Everything is all right. But is there any guarantee that you can enjoy them forever? At any moment you may be kicked out. That is not perfection. If you were guaranteed that "Whatever happy life I am preparing for in the material world will be permanent; I will never be kicked out," then your life here would be perfection. But there can never be such a guarantee. Therefore no material circumstances can be the perfection of life. The perfection of life comes when there is the guarantee of no more birth, no more death, no more old age, and no more disease. That is perfection.

And that perfection can be achieved only by Kṛṣṇa consciousness, not any material method. If we want to be eternally blissful and full of knowledge—*sac-cid-ānanda-vigraha*—then we have to take to Kṛṣṇa consciousness. There is no other way.

As Lord Kṛṣṇa says,

man-manā bhava mad-bhakto mad-yājī māṁ namaskuru
mām evaiṣyasi yuktvaivam ātmānaṁ mat-parāyaṇaḥ

"Always think of Me, become My devotee, offer obeisances unto Me, and worship Me. Without any doubt you shall come to Me." Simply four things. Is it very difficult to think of Kṛṣṇa, worship Him, become His devotee, and offer obeisances to Him? It is not difficult, as we are showing daily in our temples all over the world. We are thinking of Kṛṣṇa by chanting the Hare Kṛṣṇa *mantra.* We are offering obeisances to the Deity and at least trying to become His devotees. And we are worshiping the Lord with fruits, flowers, incense, and so on. None of this is difficult. Anyone can collect a flower, a fruit, or a little water and offer it to Kṛṣṇa.

Then where is the difficulty? The difficulty is our obstinacy. If one is obstinate, then becoming Kṛṣṇa conscious is very difficult.

Human life is meant for worshiping Kṛṣṇa. Narottama Dāsa Ṭhākura sings, *hari hari viphale janama goṅāinu:* "My life is spoiled." Why? *Manuṣya-janama pāiyā rādhā-kṛṣṇa nā bhajiyā jāniyā śuniyā viṣa khāinu:* "Having attained a human birth, I failed to worship Rādhā-Kṛṣṇa and so have knowingly drunk poison."

We are trying to stop people from drinking poison. The Kṛṣṇa consciousness movement is for everyone's benefit. It is the topmost humanitarian movement to make everyone happy, to make everyone immortal, to make everyone peaceful, to make everyone wise.

Kṛṣṇa says that one who does not surrender to Him is *narādhama,* "the lowest of mankind."

"Oh, how is he *narādhama*? He is an M.A., a Ph.D., a Dh.C., a Th.C. How is he *narādhama*?"

Māyayāpahṛta-jñāna. His knowledge has no value because he does not know Kṛṣṇa. These M.A.'s and Ph.D.'s will not help you. Kṛṣṇa says, "One who does not worship Me has no knowledge." Why? Because if one remains obstinately averse to surrendering to God, what is the value of his knowledge? He has no knowledge.

Therefore Kṛṣṇa says, *bahūnāṁ janmanām ante jñānavān māṁ prapadyate:* After many, many births of struggling to cultivate knowledge, one who is actually wise surrenders to Kṛṣṇa: "My dear Lord Kṛṣṇa, for so long I had forgotten You, not knowing that my only business is to surrender to You. But today I surrender. Please protect me." That is intelligence.

And the moment you surrender, you are protected. Lord Kṛṣṇa says,

sarva-dharmān parityajya mām ekaṁ śaraṇaṁ vraja
ahaṁ tvāṁ sarva-pāpebhyo mokṣayiṣyāmi mā śucaḥ

"Abandon all varieties of religion and just surrender unto Me. I shall deliver you from all sinful reactions. Do not fear." The Lord also promises, *kaunteya pratijānīhi na me bhaktaḥ praṇaśyati:* "My devotee never perishes."

The Kṛṣṇa consciousness movement is trying to make fools and rascals and sinful men wise. And actually it is happening. *Pāpī tāpī yata chilo, hari-nāme uddhārilo, tāra sākṣī jagāi mādhāi*. You want evidence? Look at Jagāi and Mādhāi. Caitanya Mahāprabhu delivered two sinful brothers named Jagāi and Mādhāi. Now you can see how strong is Caitanya Mahāprabhu's movement. Many thousands of Jagāis and Mādhāis are being delivered.

Caitanya Mahāprabhu's movement is greater than Caitanya Mahāprabhu. Caitanya Mahāprabhu personally delivered Jagāi and Mādhāi, but now, by His movement, thousands of Jagāis and Mādhāis are being delivered. This is the practical evidence.

And Lord Caitanya's process is very easy. It is not very difficult. Anyone can take to it. But if we knowingly take poison, who can protect us?

We appeal to everyone to take to the Kṛṣṇa consciousness movement and chant the Hare Kṛṣṇa *mantra*. Even if you cannot give up your bad habits and sinful activities at once, still take to the chanting of the Hare Kṛṣṇa *mantra*, and before long you will become purified and your life will be glorious.

Thank you very much.

Joy Beyond False Boundaries

Chanting the holy names of God in congregation raises us to pure spiritual consciousness—a state of joyful awareness of God that transcends all petty prejudices and material distinctions. Here Śrīla Prabhupāda explains the value of this chanting for the modern world. (November 1968, Los Angeles)

brahma-bhūtaḥ prasannātmā na śocati na kāṅkṣati
samaḥ sarveṣu bhūteṣu mad-bhaktiṁ labhate parām

"One who is thus transcendentally situated at once realizes the Supreme Brahman and becomes fully joyful. He never laments or desires to have anything. He is equally disposed toward every living entity. In that state he attains pure devotional service unto Me [Kṛṣṇa]" (*Bhagavad-gītā* 18.54).

Kṛṣṇa consciousness is simply full of bliss, because it is the stage one reaches after attaining liberation from all material miseries. This is called the *brahma-bhūta* stage. One feels just like a person who has been suffering in prison for many years and is suddenly given his freedom. How much delight he feels! Similarly, one who attains the *brahma-bhūta* stage immediately becomes joyful.

And what is the nature of that joyfulness? *Na śocati:* even if one suffers great loss, one does not lament. And *na kāṅkṣati:* one feels no hankering for big profit. Also, in that stage one sees all living entities on the same platform of spiritual identity. In another place the *Bhagavad-gītā* says, *paṇḍitaḥ sama-darśinaḥ:* "When a person is learned he sees everyone on the same level of spiritual identity." At this stage, Kṛṣṇa consciousness actually begins (*mad-bhaktiṁ labhate parām*). So Kṛṣṇa consciousness is the activity of the living entity in the liberated stage.

Everyone is trying to get liberation from material pangs. Those who follow Buddhist philosophy are trying to get liberation from material miseries by reaching *nirvāṇa*. *Nirvāṇa* means "the stage when everything is extinguished." The Buddhists want to make everything void; they want to make all material varieties zero. That is the sum and substance of Buddhist philosophy. And Māyāvāda [impersonalistic] philosophy is more or less similar. It is a second edition of Buddhist philosophy. The Buddhists want to make everything zero without life, and the Māyāvādī philosophers say, "Yes, we should make the material varieties zero, but keep life." That is their mistake. Where there is life, there must be variety; life without variety is not possible. This is the defect of Māyāvāda philosophy.

Suppose a patient is very much disturbed and he asks his physician, "Please stop my disturbance! Kill me! Kill me!" Sometimes people who are suffering speak like that. "Give me some poison! Kill me! I cannot tolerate the pain!"'

The physician says, "There is no need to kill you. I shall give you a good, healthy life."

But the diseased man is so impatient: "No, I cannot tolerate. Please kill me!"

So Buddhist and Māyāvādī philosophers are like this. They think, "I want to die; I want to become zero, void." They are feeling so much frustration, so much disturbance from the material miseries, that they want to make their life zero.

Kṛṣṇa consciousness is not like that. Kṛṣṇa consciousness brings you to real life—a life of devotional activity in the liberated stage.

But it is often difficult to understand the philosophy of Kṛṣṇa consciousness. Why? That is explained in *Śrīmad-Bhāgavatam* [7.5.30]: *matir na kṛṣṇe parataḥ svato vā mitho 'bhipadyeta gṛha-vratānām. Gṛha* means "house," and *vrata* means "vow." So the *Bhāgavatam* says, "One who is too interested in maintaining a comfortable family life cannot understand the philosophy of Kṛṣṇa consciousness." Everywhere the common man is interested in attaining bodily comforts, a nice wife, a nice apartment, a nice bank balance. These things are his aspirations, and nothing more.

First of all a person is interested in his body. *Gṛha* means "house" or "living place." I am a soul, a living being, and my body is my first living place. The body is also a *gṛha.* But I am not the body. I may live in an apartment, but I am not the apartment. Similarly, I am living in a body, but I am not the body. This understanding is the beginning of spiritual education. Unless a person understands that he is not his body—that he is a spirit soul living *in* his body—there is no question of spiritual education, because such a person does not know how to distinguish what is spiritual from what is material.

So it is a misunderstanding to think "I am my body. I belong to my apartment. I belong to my society. I belong to my nation. I belong to my world. I belong to my universe." You may expand the idea of *gṛha,* but it is all a misunderstanding, whether you are a big leader who says, "My life is for my nation," or a common man who says, "My life is for my family," or some childlike person who says, "I am interested only in my body." People very much appreciate it when we expand our conception of self-interest from bodily welfare to family welfare, or from family welfare to community welfare, or from community welfare to national welfare, or from national welfare to the idea of universal brotherhood. But these are all bogus ideas, misconceptions.

However you may expand the *gṛha,* the defect will remain. For example, the so-called nationalists in America are packed up within the boundary of human beings: they do not expand their affection to other living entities. They believe that the human beings living in America should be given protection but that the animals need no protection. Why? The cows and other animals in America are also nationals; they should also be protected. But the nationalists have no such idea, because nationalism and all such ideas are defective and limited.

So the *Bhāgavatam* says that as long as a person is interested in keeping himself within the boundary of some limited conception of life he cannot understand Kṛṣṇa consciousness, or God consciousness. *Matir na kṛṣṇe parataḥ svato vā. Svataḥ* means "by one's personal mental speculation." Many philosophers are thinking they will reach the Absolute Truth by mental speculation. And *parataḥ. Parataḥ* means "from authorities"—from the spiritual master, the scriptures, or other authoritative sources of knowledge. Our principle is to receive knowledge from the spiritual master. But suppose somebody thinks, "I am American. Why should I hear from a spiritual master who is Hindu?" Such a person will not be able to understand the teachings of Kṛṣṇa consciousness. So those who are *gṛha-vratānām,* determined to remain within a limited conception of life, cannot understand Kṛṣṇa consciousness—either by their own mental efforts or by taking help from authorities.

Next the *Bhāgavatam* uses the word *mithaḥ,* which means "taking part in a great assembly." A good example is the United Nations. The United Nations has been trying to bring world peace for the last twenty, twenty-five years. So why has it not been possible? Because the representatives at the United Nations have a limited conception of life. They think, "I am my body, which was born in such-and-such a nation." The basic principle is wrong, the conception of life is wrong, and therefore the United Nations has failed to bring peace in the world.

Now, why are people limited by a poor conception of life? The *Bhāgavatam* says, *adānta-gobhiḥ.* The limited conception of life is caused by unbridled senses. Everyone wants to satisfy his senses, or the senses of his countrymen. So although a man may go to the assembly of the United Nations, he keeps his identity as American or German or Russian or Indian, and he thinks, "My nation shall be happy in such-and-such a way." The Indian is thinking like this, the American is thinking like this, the Russian is thinking like this. But if they keep themselves in that limited conception of life, what benefit will they derive? They will simply talk and waste time. That's all. Only when one goes outside these limited conceptions of life and reaches the *brahma-bhūta* stage can one have real peace.

Next the *Bhāgavatam* describes the position of someone

with uncontrolled senses: *punaḥ punaś carvita-carvaṇānām. Carvita-carvaṇa* means "chewing the chewed." Suppose something is chewed and then thrown away in the street. If somebody comes and again chews that thrown-away article, he cannot get any juice out of it. Similarly, we may try repeatedly to enjoy our senses in this material world, but all our efforts must end in frustration.

We may make so many plans, but because all our plans are on the platform of sense gratification, our whole existence is limited to the four activities of animal life: eating, sleeping, mating, and defending. That's all. Animals and men have these four activities in common. The only extra qualification of man is that he can come to understand Kṛṣṇa, or God. That is his special qualification. But because people keep themselves within the limits of sense gratification, they come again and again to the same platform of eating, sleeping, mating, and defending. Therefore they remain without Kṛṣṇa consciousness.

So, the secret of how to become Kṛṣṇa conscious is that we should not limit ourselves to a narrow conception of life. How is that possible? We must understand, "I am an eternal servant of Kṛṣṇa, or God." That is Kṛṣṇa consciousness.

Now, one may ask, "If understanding Kṛṣṇa is the goal of life, why do people keep themselves within the limit of sense gratification?" That question is answered in the next verse of *Śrīmad-Bhāgavatam* [7.5.31]: *na te viduḥ svārtha-gatiṁ hi viṣṇuṁ durāśayā ye bahir-artha-māninaḥ.* This is a very important verse. It says that foolish persons do not know that Viṣṇu, or Kṛṣṇa, is the ultimate goal of their life because they are entrapped by the consciousness of enjoying material nature. Everyone is eager to look after his self-interest, but foolish people do not know what their real self-interest is. They are thinking, "Working hard in the material way of life will give me ultimate pleasure, ultimate satisfaction. That is my ultimate goal." The scientist, the politician—everyone is making his own plan to reach ultimate satisfaction. And how will they fulfill that plan? By manipulating nature, Kṛṣṇa's external energy (*bahir-artha-māninaḥ*).

We are preaching Kṛṣṇa consciousness, but most people are not interested. Had I been an expert in a new kind of technology, or in teaching an improvement in electronics, thousands of people would be coming to hear me. Because I would have been dealing with the ingredients of the external energy, people would have thought, "This technological knowledge will give me happiness." That is *durāśayā,* a useless hope. The *Bhāgavatam* says this kind of material advancement is useless. It will not give you any happiness. But people are foolishly hoping it will.

Now the *Bhāgavatam* says, *andhā yathāndhair upanīyamānāḥ.* This means that those people who are hoping for happiness through material advancement are spiritually blind. They do not know the goal of life, and their leaders also do not know the goal of life. People are thinking that with the change of some politician something new will be done and they will be happy. Now there is an advertisement: "America needs Nixon now." People are thinking, "When Nixon will be president instead of Johnson, we shall be happy." [*Laughter.*] But from which stock are this Johnson and Nixon coming? The source of supply is the same. If the source of supply is the same, what is the use of replacing Johnson with Nixon or Nixon with Johnson?

The leaders are spiritually blind: they do not know the ultimate goal of life. If the people are blind and their leaders are also blind, what will be the result? If a blind man leads one hundred other blind men across the street, certainly there will be some accident. But if the leader can see, he can lead hundreds and thousands of men safely.

Now the *Bhāgavatam* explains, *te 'pīśa-tantryām urudāmni baddhāḥ:* "Both the blind leaders and their blind followers are very tightly bound by the strong ropes of material nature." The leaders promise, "My dear citizens, my dear countrymen, the country needs me at the present moment. If you give me your vote, I shall give you all comforts, all solutions." But all these leaders are tightly bound up by the laws of God, the laws of nature. You see? If your hands and legs are tightly bound, how can you work? The leaders do not know that they are under the stringent control of the laws of nature. Suppose there is a heavy earthquake, or suppose the Atlantic Ocean and the Pacific Ocean mix together. Then how can you check the laws of nature? Your hands and legs are tightly bound by nature's laws. You cannot check them. So how can blind leaders, who are so tightly bound up by the laws of nature, lead people to the ultimate goal of life? The ultimate goal of life is God, or Kṛṣṇa, but the leaders are enamored by the glitter of this material nature. So they cannot lead us to Kṛṣṇa.

Then what is the solution to our problem? If it is not possible to attain Kṛṣṇa consciousness by speculation, by assembly meetings, or by deriving knowledge from authoritative sources, then how is it to be attained? How can the goal of life be reached?

The next verse of *Śrīmad-Bhāgavatam* [7.5.32] answers this question:

naiṣāṁ matis tāvad urukramāṅghriṁ
spṛśaty anarthāpagamo yad-arthaḥ
mahīyasāṁ pāda-rajo-'bhiṣekaṁ
niṣkiñcanānāṁ na vṛṇīta yāvat

One cannot fix his mind on the lotus feet of Kṛṣṇa unless one has the opportunity of touching the dust of the lotus feet of a person who has given up all material hankerings (*niṣkiñcanānām*) and who has dedicated his life cent percent to Kṛṣṇa (*mahīyasām*). When one comes in touch with such a person, by his grace one can attain Kṛṣṇa consciousness—not by any other method. One must approach a bona fide spiritual master and by his mercy, by his grace, receive Kṛṣṇa consciousness. And as soon as a person receives initiation into Kṛṣṇa consciousness, he feels spiritual satisfaction, and his liberation from material entanglement begins. Then, as he makes further and further progress, his life becomes sublime.

The first benefit of Kṛṣṇa consciousness is that as soon as a person comes in touch with Kṛṣṇa he immediately gives up all the unwholesome activities of material existence. In fact, we can test if someone is in contact with Kṛṣṇa by seeing how free he is from sinful activity. For example (not a very gigantic example—a very small one), take our students. As soon as they are initiated into Kṛṣṇa consciousness, they immediately give up so many sinful activities. The basic activities of sinful life are illicit sex, intoxication, meat-eating, and gambling. It is very difficult for people to give up all these habits, especially in the Western countries. But my students are giving them up very easily.

In 1935 one of my Godbrothers went to London and met the Marquis of Zetland, a man from Scotland. He was very interested in Indian philosophy. (He had previously been the governor of Bengal, and in my youth I had met him; he had come to my college.) So the marquis inquired from my Godbrother, Goswami Bannerjee: "Bannerjee, can you make me a *brāhmaṇa*?"

Bannerjee said, "Why not? Yes, we can make you a *brāhmaṇa,* but you have to follow four rules. You must give up illicit sex, intoxication, meat-eating, and gambling. Then you can become a *brāhmaṇa*."

"Oh, that is impossible."

You see? The Marquis of Zetland was such a big personality—he was interested in philosophy, he held a high government position, he was a responsible man—yet he flatly denied that he could give up these four sinful habits. But our students, hundreds of boys and girls who are coming to Kṛṣṇa consciousness, are giving up these habits very easily. And they don't feel any inconvenience. This is the first benefit of Kṛṣṇa consciousness: In the very beginning one is finished with all sinful activity.

How can our students give up these things? Because they are feeling spiritual satisfaction in Kṛṣṇa consciousness: Our students can sit down before the Deity and chant Hare Kṛṣṇa for twenty-four hours. Bring any student of any other yoga society and ask him to sit down for five hours. He'll fail; he'll be so restless. These so-called yoga societies simply teach their students some official meditation: fifteen minutes to a half hour of closing the eyes and murmuring something. But our students are engaged in Kṛṣṇa consciousness twenty-four hours a day. Anyone may come and ask them how they are feeling. Unless they feel some spiritual satisfaction, how can they give up everything and simply serve Kṛṣṇa?

Now, one may ask, "Suppose a person takes up Kṛṣṇa consciousness out of sentiment but he cannot complete the process. What is his position?" This question is also answered in *Śrīmad-Bhāgavatam* [1.5.17]:

tyaktvā sva-dharmaṁ caraṇāmbujaṁ harer
bhajann apakvo 'tha patet tato yadi
yatra kva vābhadram abhūd amuṣya kiṁ
ko vārtha āpto 'bhajatāṁ sva-dharmataḥ

The word *sva-dharma* means "specific duty." Everyone has some specific duty or occupation. So somebody may give up his specific duty and begin practicing Kṛṣṇa consciousness. All of my students were engaged in something else, but all of a sudden they gave it up and joined the Kṛṣṇa consciousness movement. So, anyone may do this. After hearing some lectures on Kṛṣṇa consciousness, someone may decide, "Now I shall begin Kṛṣṇa consciousness." So he gives up his occupation and begins chanting Hare Kṛṣṇa and following the other devotional principles. But all of a sudden he gives them up. For some reason, because of some unfortunate circumstances, he cannot prosecute Kṛṣṇa consciousness nicely and he gives it up. So the *Bhāgavatam* says that even if one gives up Kṛṣṇa consciousness because of immaturity, still there is no loss, because he will take it up again in the next life.

But then the *Bhāgavatam* says, *ko vārtha āpto 'bhajatāṁ sva-dharmataḥ:* "What profit is there for someone who very steadily engages in his occupational duty but is without any Kṛṣṇa consciousness?" He is simply a loser, because he does not know the aim of his life. But if a person takes to Kṛṣṇa consciousness even for a few days, if he gets the injection of Kṛṣṇa consciousness, in his next life he'll take it up again. So he's not a loser. That one injection will someday make him perfect in Kṛṣṇa consciousness, and he's sure to go back to Godhead.

So execute Kṛṣṇa consciousness, and try to spread Kṛṣṇa consciousness as far as possible. Rest assured, your efforts will not go in vain. They will *not* go in vain. Kṛṣṇa will reward you abundantly.

Thank you very much.

The Mercy of Lord Caitanya

More than five hundred years ago, Kṛṣṇa came to this world as Lord Caitanya to freely distribute love of Godhead through the chanting of the Hare Kṛṣṇa mantra. *In this lecture Śrīla Prabhupāda describes how Lord Caitanya's unlimited mercy can bring true unity among nations. (March of 1975, Atlanta, Georgia)*

namo mahā-vadānyāya kṛṣṇa-prema-pradāya te
kṛṣṇāya kṛṣṇa-caitanya-nāmne gaura-tviṣe namaḥ

"O most munificent incarnation! You are Kṛṣṇa Himself appearing as Śrī Kṛṣṇa Caitanya Mahāprabhu. You have assumed the golden color of Śrīmatī Rādhārāṇī, and You are widely distributing pure love of Kṛṣṇa. We offer our respectful obeisances unto You" (*Caitanya-caritāmṛta*, *Madhya-līlā* 19.53).

Caitanya Mahāprabhu wanted to preach love of Kṛṣṇa, love of God, not only in India but all over the world. Different religions have many different names of God, and in the Vedic scriptures there are many demigods and incarnations of God. But Kṛṣṇa is the original name of God. As said in the *Śrīmad-Bhāgavatam* [1.3.28], *ete cāṁśa-kalāḥ puṁsaḥ kṛṣṇas tu bhagavān svayam.* There is a list of incarnations, and at the conclusion of the list the *Bhāgavatam* says, "In this long list there are many names, but Kṛṣṇa is the original Supreme Personality of Godhead."

God is not like us—He can expand Himself. Even some yogis (not these ordinary, third-class yogis, but those who have attained yogic perfection) can expand their bodies up to at most eight times. There are instances of yogis doing that. So if an ordinary yogi can do that, just imagine how much potency the Supreme Lord has for expanding Himself!

In the *Bhagavad-gītā* [18.61] Kṛṣṇa says, *īśvaraḥ sarva-bhūtānāṁ hṛd-deśe 'rjuna tiṣṭhati:* "My dear Arjuna, the Supreme Lord is situated in every living being's heart." Just imagine how many living entities there are! They cannot be counted. There are many millions of trillions, but even "millions of trillions" is insignificant. There is no counting them. Yet they are all part and parcel of God, and He is living within the heart of each one of them. This is the unlimited potency of the Supreme Personality of Godhead.

Consider the sunshine, the sun globe, and the sun-god. The sun-god is within the sun globe, and the inhabitants of the sun globe are all luminous. On account of their bodies' glowing, the whole sun planet is glowing. And on account of the sun planet's glowing, the sunshine reaches us from ninety-three million miles away, and we perceive heat and light. The sun is an ordinary material thing, but it has such great power.

Now, if an ordinary thing like the sun globe is so powerful, how much more powerful must be the Supreme Personality of Godhead! We say, "God is almighty, all-powerful," but we have no idea what is meant by "all-powerful." We think, "I am somewhat powerful, so God may be ten times as powerful as I am." Somebody else may say "twenty times." "All right, let us compromise—fifty times." [*Laughter*].

This kind of speculation is like the frog's speculation within the well. Once there was a frog within a well, and one of his friends came to him and said, "My dear friend, I have seen a vast mass of water, the Atlantic Ocean."

"What is that Atlantic Ocean?"

"It is vast."

"How vast? Is it ten times bigger than this well? Or twenty times? Come!" [*Laughter*.]

"No, no, it is very, very vast."

So, the rascal speculation about God is like the speculation of the frog about the Atlantic Ocean. These mundane philosophers and scientists are thinking of God in that way. Dr. Frog's philosophy will not help you understand what God is.

Śrī Caitanya Mahāprabhu's preaching was to distribute love of God. This human life is especially meant for understanding what God is and loving Him. That's all. This is our only business. The cats and dogs and other lower animals—if you preach to them about Kṛṣṇa consciousness, they will not understand. But human beings can understand. For example, this Kṛṣṇa consciousness movement is being spread all over the world, and as you can see, here in your country people are understanding. That is the special advantage of human life.

One Christian priest in Boston was astonished to see our devotees. He issued a leaflet saying, "These Hare Kṛṣṇa boys are our boys. Before they joined this movement they did not care to see us or come to the church, but now they are mad after God." So this movement is certified by a Christian priest.

And actually, you can see the potency of Lord Caitanya's movement. I am a poor Indian; I came to America with forty rupees. I had no money to bribe these young people. [*Laughter.*] But now they are mad after God. It is practical. Now if you try to bribe them to leave this movement, they will not go.

So, what is the intoxication? These boys and girls have given up all intoxication, but they are now "intoxicated" with "Hare Kṛṣṇa, Hare Kṛṣṇa." This is the mercy of Lord Caitanya Mahāprabhu. A draft-board officer came to see one of our centers. He said, "What is the facility you have given these boys who have joined the Hare Kṛṣṇa movement? It must be much easier than the army." But when he investigated, he saw that these boys and girls are prohibited from engaging in illicit sex, intoxication, meat-eating, and gambling. So he concluded that this movement is actually *harder* than the army. The army does not make these restrictions, which are very, very difficult to follow. But by the mercy of Caitanya Mahāprabhu, these boys and girls are following them.

Every human being should accept the mercy of Śrī Caitanya Mahāprabhu. That is the purport of the verse Rūpa Gosvāmī offered to Lord Caitanya upon seeing Him: *namo mahā-vadānyāya*. "You are the most munificent incarnation of God." Why? "You are distributing *kṛṣṇa-prema,* love of

God. People do not know what God is, yet You are distributing love of Godhead."

Ordinarily one cannot love anybody unless he knows the other party very well. Only then is there a question of love. If you and I live ten thousand miles apart, there is no question of love. For love there must be intimacy.

So, to understand God is very difficult. In the *Bhagavad-gītā* [7.3], Kṛṣṇa says,

manuṣyāṇāṁ sahasreṣu kaścid yatati siddhaye
yatatām api siddhānāṁ kaścin māṁ vetti tattvataḥ

"Out of many millions of persons, one is interested in making his life perfect. And out of all those who are actually perfect, hardly one knows Me as I am."

Perfection does not mean that I can eat whatever I like, without any restriction. Or that I have a very nice car, a very nice apartment, and a big bank balance. This is not perfection, because I remain under the grip of the laws of material nature. *Prakṛteḥ kriyamāṇāni guṇaiḥ karmāṇi sarvaśaḥ*. The material nature is controlling me.

How is the material nature controlling? She has a machine made of the three modes of nature. *Kāraṇaṁ guṇa-saṅgo 'sya sad-asad-yoni-janmasu*. People are contacting these three modes of nature and thus being "infected." We know that if we contract some disease, knowingly or unknowingly, that disease will develop. This is the law of nature. Even if you do not know when or how you contracted a particular disease, that is no excuse. You must suffer.

Similarly, there are three modes of material nature one can become "infected" by—goodness, passion, and ignorance. Not knowing about this is no excuse. If in the law court you say "Your Honor, I did not know I would be punished for stealing," the magistrate or judge will not excuse you. And if the government law is so strict, you can imagine how strict are the stringent laws of material nature.

Knowingly or unknowingly, in this life we are being infected by a particular combination of the modes of material nature and thus creating our next body. There are 8,400,000 different varieties of life forms. Why? The answer is in the *Bhagavad-gītā: kāraṇaṁ guṇa-saṅgaḥ*. There are so many different species of life because each living entity is becoming infected with a particular combination of the qualities of material nature. This is going on perpetually. "Perpetually" means we do not know when this process began or when it will end. Therefore we say it is perpetual.

In this human form of life we have the great advantage of being able to study all these things—what is the living entity, how he is being infected by material nature, and how he is taking different bodies. The first thing we must understand is that we are not the body. Therefore in the very beginning of the *Bhagavad-gītā* Lord Kṛṣṇa tries to impress upon us that we are not this body but rather the owner or occupier of the body. This is His first instruction. If we understand this instruction, we can rise above the bodily platform.

Caitanya Mahāprabhu's movement is not on the bodily platform; it is on the spiritual platform. This He explained when He talked with Sanātana Gosvāmī. Sanātana asked, "What is my identity?" He was a very learned man—a minister and a *brāhmaṇa*. He knew Sanskrit and Urdu very well. Because the kingdom he lived in was Muslim, Urdu was the state language, just as during the British period the state language was English. So, Sanātana Gosvāmī was quite conversant with Urdu, Farsi, and Sanskrit. Therefore he said to Sri Caitanya Mahāprabhu, "Ordinary people address me as *paṇḍitjī,* a very learned man, but I know my position. I do not know what I am. This is my position."

Now, if you ask a big, big doctor, scientist, or philosopher, "What are you?" he will say, "I am an Indian," or "I am an American," or "I am this, I am that." Bodily designations, that's all. He is fool number one, and still he is passing as a great scientist, a great philosopher.

If one does not know himself, what is the value of his learning? One must know his own identity. Everyone is identifying with his body: "I am Hindu," "I am Muslim," "I am Christian," "I am Indian," "I am American," "I am German," "I am English." This is why so much fighting is going on. The living entity is part and parcel of God, a spiritual spark covered by a material body. For example, we are all human beings covered by different clothes. That does not mean we are essentially different. We are one as human beings, as inhabitants of this earth. But due to our different bodily dress, I am thinking you are my enemy, and you are thinking I am your enemy.

The *Bhāgavatam's* conclusion is *yasyātma-buddhiḥ kuṇape tri-dhātuke sva-dhiḥ kalatrādiṣu bhauma-ijya-dhiḥ . . . sa eva go-kharaḥ:* "Anyone who is identifying himself with his body and family, and also with the land his body has taken birth in, is no better than an ass or a cow." Everyone is thinking, "This land of my birth is worshipable." And from this mentality comes nationalism or this "ism" or that "ism." But no one thinks, "How long shall I be allowed to occupy this body and this land?" This is ignorance.

So, Śrī Caitanya Mahāprabhu's movement starts from the understanding that we are spirit souls, eternal servants of Kṛṣṇa. This teaching is the same as Kṛṣṇa's in the *Bhagavad-gītā*. There the Lord says, *sarva-dharmān parityajya mām ekaṁ śaraṇaṁ vraja:* "Give up your so-called man-made duties, or *dharmas,* and just surrender unto Me." This is real *dharma,* or religion—to surrender to God.

God is one. He is neither Hindu nor Muslim nor Christian. The Vedic injunction is *ekaṁ brahma dvitīyaṁ nāsti:* "God is one; He cannot be two." So whether you are Hindu, Muslim, or Christian, God is one. This is to be understood.

Kṛṣṇa consciousness is the science of God. Try to understand scientifically what you are and what God is and what religion is. That is Caitanya Mahāprabhu's teaching. He begins His teachings to Sanātana Gosvāmī by saying *jīvera 'svarūpa' haya—kṛṣṇera 'nitya-dāsa':* "Every living being is an eternal servant of God." This is religion. Religion does not mean stamping oneself as a Hindu, a Muslim, or a Christian.

No. Religion means to know that God is great and that we are subordinate to Him and maintained by Him. This is religion. If anyone simply knows these things—that God is great and we are subordinate, and that our duty is to abide by the orders of God—he is religious.

Unity can be established on the spiritual platform, not on the bodily platform. The United Nations is trying to unite the nations of the world, but every year the number of flags is increasing. This kind of so-called unity will never be successful. The United Nations was established many years ago to bring unity among nations. So, what has it done? It has not done anything, nor can it do anything.

If you want to be united, you have to be united on the spiritual platform. And what is that spiritual platform? The spiritual platform means to understand thoroughly that God is great, that we are subordinate, and that God is maintaining us. All the property everywhere belongs to God, and while we can use our father's property as much as we require, we should not take more than we need and stock it.

The birds are a good example. If you put a bag of rice in the street, the birds will come and eat a few grains and go away. But if you put, say, one thousand bags of wheat in the street and declare that anyone can take them, there will be a fight. Everyone will try to take as much as he can carry. This is human civilization: "Oh, there is so much wheat. Let me take as much as possible and stock it for tomorrow or the day after tomorrow. Let me stock it for my son, my grandson, and my great-grandson." [*Laughter*.]

This foolishness is going on because of a lack of spiritual consciousness. As stated in the *Vedas, īśāvāsyam idaṁ sarvam:* "Everything belongs to God." The food belongs to God, the mine belongs to God, the ocean belongs to God, the land belongs to God, the air belongs to God—everything belongs to God. So we should feel obliged to God that he has given us so much for our maintenance. We should take as much as we need and use as much as possible in His service. This is Kṛṣṇa consciousness.

Kṛṣṇa consciousness is actually perfect communism. The communists think in terms of the human beings within the state, but a Kṛṣṇa conscious person thinks in terms of all living beings. In the *Bhāgavatam* it is stated that a householder, before taking his lunch, should call out on the street: "If anyone is hungry, please come to my place and eat!" And he should see that in his household even the lizard does not go hungry. Even a snake should not hungry. This is the Vedic principle, God consciousness. The householder thinks, "Somehow or other some living entity has taken a snake's body. So at my house why should he remain hungry? Let me give him some food." Nobody likes snakes, but in the scripture it is said that one should see to it that even a snake does not go hungry.

Of course, this is a very high ideal, but it is the complete ideal of real communism. It is not that national leaders should be concerned only with human beings. The definition of native is "one who takes birth in a particular nation." So, the cow is also a native. Then why should the cow be slaughtered? The cow is giving milk and the bull is working for you, and then you slaughter them? What is this philosophy? In the Christian religion it is clearly stated, "Thou shalt not kill." Yet most of the slaughterhouses are in the Christian countries.

This is all a misunderstanding of spiritual life. Every animal should be given protection. That is the Vedic idea. Otherwise, by killing, killing, killing, you become entangled in sinful activities. Therefore now the women are killing their own children in the womb. This is going on.

We cannot be happy in this way, because we shall become more and more entangled in sinful actions and their resultant reactions. Then we will have to take various types of bodies, perpetually.

Therefore, we have begun this Kṛṣṇa consciousness movement. By taking advantage of this movement, people can awaken to God consciousness, stop sinful activities, and become purified. Without becoming purified, one cannot understand God. It is not possible. As Kṛṣṇa says in the *Bhagavad-gītā* [7.28],

yeṣāṁ tv anta-gataṁ pāpaṁ janānāṁ puṇya-karmaṇām
te dvandva-moha-nirmuktā bhajante māṁ dṛḍha-vratāḥ

"One who is completely free from sinful life can take to devotional service with great determination."

That is why we have prescribed four regulative principles: no illicit sex, no meat-eating, no gambling, and no intoxication. Especially in your country, America, you have so many nice vegetables, fruits, grains, and milk products. So why should you kill the cow? You have taken our *prasādam* feasts. How delicious they are! So why kill the cow?

Sometimes people argue that vegetables also have life. Yes, we admit this. But that is why we eat only *prasādam,* food offered to Kṛṣṇa before being eaten. Whatever Kṛṣṇa leaves, we take. This is our process. We don't take directly. So, while the vegetables have life, Kṛṣṇa says, *patraṁ puṣpaṁ phalaṁ toyaṁ yo me bhaktyā prayacchati tad ahaṁ . . . aśnāmi:* "If one lovingly offers Me a leaf, a flower, a fruit, or water, I will accept it." Then there is no sin in eating the vegetables.

We have invited Kṛṣṇa as our guest, and He has consented to come here. So we must offer Him the foods He wants. That is proper etiquette. If some respectable guest comes to your house, you should ask him, "What would you like to eat, sir?" Whatever he asks for, you have to supply. That is the real way of receiving a guest.

So Kṛṣṇa says, "Give Me food among these items: fruits, vegetables, grains, and milk products. And that also with devotion, not neglectfully. Then I will accept it." Therefore we prepare hundreds of items with these ingredients and offer them to Kṛṣṇa, and you can also do that. They are all delicious and full of vitamins. Then why should you unnecessarily kill the poor animals and become vicious and sinful?

This is Kṛṣṇa Caitanya Mahāprabhu's teaching: Live

peacefully, be a gentleman, chant Hare Kṛṣṇa, realize God, and make your life happy in this world and the next. He wanted this teaching spread to every town, every city, every village in the world. And the Hare Kṛṣṇa movement is just trying to serve Lord Caitanya Mahāprabhu. You can see how beneficial this Kṛṣṇa consciousness is. Please don't be blind, but try to consider it a little liberally, without any sophistry or prejudice. Try to understand the philosophy of Caitanya Mahāprabhu and be happy.

Thank you very much.

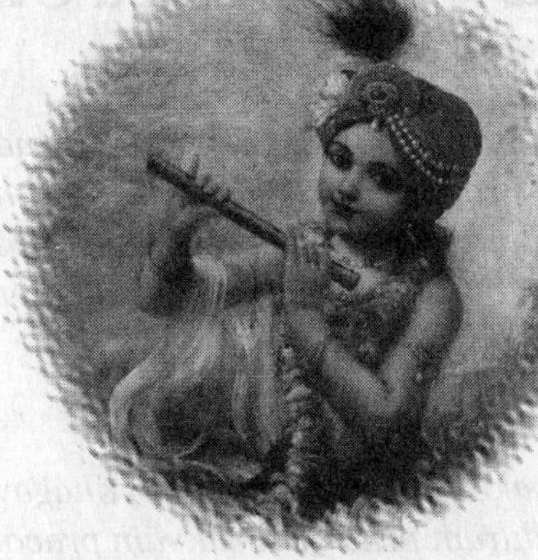

3. The Spiritual Master

Who Is a Guru, And Why We Need One

"One who is inquisitive to understand the ultimate goal of life must approach a proper guru," says Śrīla Prabhupāda in this lecture given in Mumbai, India, in November of 1974. Then he explains what that ultimate goal is, how that approach must be made, and who is the proper guru.

sūta uvāca
dvaipāyana-sakhas tv evaṁ maitreyo bhagavāṁs tathā
prāhedaṁ viduraṁ prīta ānvīkṣikyāṁ pracoditaḥ

"Śrī Sūta Gosvāmī said: 'The most powerful sage Maitreya was a friend of Vyāsadeva's. Being encouraged and pleased by Vidura's inquiry about transcendental knowledge, Maitreya spoke as follows" [*Śrīmad-Bhāgavatam* 3.25.4].

This is the process for getting transcendental knowledge: to approach the proper person, the guru, and submissively hear from him. *Tad viddhi praṇipātena paripraśnena sevayā.* Although the process is very easy, one must know the process and follow it. For example, suppose your typewriter is not working. Then you have to go to the proper person, someone who knows how to fix it. He will immediately tighten a screw or fix something else, and it works. But if you go to a vegetable seller for repairing the machine, that will not be good. He does not know the process. He may know how to sell vegetables, but that doesn't matter: he does not know how to repair a typewriter.

Therefore the Vedic injunction is *tad-vijñānārthaṁ sa gurum evābhigacchet*. If you want to learn transcendental knowledge (*tad-vijñāna*), you must approach a guru. Actually, human life is meant for understanding transcendental knowledge, not material knowledge. Material knowledge all pertains to the body. A medical practitioner may have so much knowledge of the mechanical arrangement of the body, but he has no knowledge of the spirit soul. Therefore he cannot help you fulfill the goal of your life.

The body is a machine made by nature (*yantrārūḍhāni māyayā*). For those who are very much attached to this machine, the meditative yoga system is recommended. In this system one learns to perform some gymnastics and concentrate the mind, so that eventually the mind may be focused on Lord Viṣṇu. The real purpose is to understand Viṣṇu, the Supreme Lord. So the yoga system is more or less a mechanical arrangement. But the *bhakti* system is above this mechanical arrangement. Therefore *bhakti* begins with the search for *tad-vijñāna,* spiritual knowledge.

So, if you want to understand spiritual knowledge, you have to approach a guru. One meaning of the word *guru* is "weighty." Therefore the guru is one who is "heavy" with knowledge. And what is that knowledge? That is explained in the *Kaṭhopaniṣad: śrotriyaṁ brahma-niṣṭham. Śrotriyaṁ* means "one who has received knowledge by hearing the *Vedas,* the *śruti,*" and *brahma-niṣṭham* indicates one who has realized Brahman, or rather Parabrahman, Bhagavān, the Supreme Personality of Godhead. That is the guru's qualification.

One must hear from those who are in the line of preceptorial succession, or disciplic succession. As Lord Kṛṣṇa says in the *Bhagavad-gītā, evaṁ paramparā-prāptam.* If one wants standard transcendental knowledge, not upstart knowledge, one must received it from the *paramparā* system, the disciplic succession. Another meaning of the word *śrotriyam* mentioned above is "one who has heard from a guru in the disciplic succession." And the result of this hearing will be *brahma-niṣṭham,* "He is firmly fixed in the service of the Supreme Personality of Godhead." He has no other business. These are the two main qualifications of a bona fide guru. He does not need to be a very learned scholar with an M.A., B.A., or Ph.D. No. He simply needs to have heard from the authority in disciplic succession and be fixed in devotional service. This is our system.

In the verse under discussion we see that Vidura was hearing from Maitreya Ṛṣi and that Maitreya was very much pleased (*viduraṁ prītaḥ*). Unless you satisfy your guru very nicely, you cannot get the right knowledge. That is natural. If you receive your guru properly and give him a very nice place where he can sit comfortably, and if he is pleased with your behavior, then he will speak very frankly and very freely, which will be beneficial for you. This is the case with Vidura and Maitreya: Maitreya Ṛṣi was very much pleased with Vidura, and thus Maitreya imparted instructions to him.

Lord Kṛṣṇa recommends the same procedure in the *Bhagavad-gītā: tad viddhi praṇipātena paripraśnena sevayā.* "One must offer obeisances to the guru, inquire from him, and serve him." If you simply go and ask the spiritual master questions in a challenging spirit but do not accept his instructions and do not render service, then you're wasting your time. The word used here is *praṇipātena,* "offering obeisances with no reservation." So reception of transcendental knowledge is based on this *praṇipāta*. That is why Kṛṣṇa says later, *sarva-dharmān parityajya mām ekaṁ śaraṇaṁ vraja*: "Give up everything else and just surrender unto Me." Just as we have to surrender to Kṛṣṇa, we have to surrender to Kṛṣṇa's representative, the spiritual master.

The guru is the external representative of Kṛṣṇa. The internal guru is Kṛṣṇa Himself (*īśvaraḥ sarva-bhūtānāṁ hṛd-deśe 'rjuna tiṣṭhati*). It is not that Kṛṣṇa is only in Goloka Vṛndāvana, the spiritual world. He is everywhere, within every atom and within everyone's heart (*goloka eva nivasaty akhilātma-bhūtaḥ*). The manifestation of Kṛṣṇa in the heart is the Paramātmā, or Supersoul. I am an *ātmā,* an individual soul, you are an *ātmā*. We are both situated locally—you are situated within your body, and I am situated within my body. But the Paramātmā is situated everywhere. That is the difference between the *ātmā* and the Paramātmā. Some people think there is no difference between the *ātmā* and the Paramātmā, but there is a difference. They are one in the sense that both of them are cognizant living entities, but they are different in that the Paramātmā is all-pervading and the *ātmā* is localized. Kṛṣṇa confirms this in the *Bhagavad-gītā: kṣetra-jñaṁ cāpi māṁ viddhi sarva-kṣetreṣu bhārata.* "Besides the individual soul in each body, I am also present as the Supersoul." The word *kṣetra-jña* means "the knower of the *kṣetra,* or body." So I am the knower or occupier of my body. The body is just like a house, with a tenant and a landlord. The tenant may occupy the house, but the landlord is the proprietor. Similarly, we *ātmās* are simply tenants of our bodies; we are not the proprietor. The proprietor is the Paramātmā. And when the proprietor says, "Get out of this house, get out of this body" you have to leave your body, and that is called death. This is Vedic knowledge.

So, one who is inquisitive to understand the ultimate goal of life must approach a proper guru. An ordinary man interested in the bodily comforts of life doesn't require a guru. Today, however, a guru is generally taken to mean someone who can give you some bodily remedy. People will approach some so-called saintly person and ask, "Mahātmājī, I am suffering from this disease." "Yes, I have a *mantra* that will cure you." That sort of guru is accepted—to cure some disease or give some wealth. No. Lord Kṛṣṇa says in the *Bhagavad-gītā* [4.34],

tad viddhi praṇipātena paripraśnena sevayā
upadekṣyanti te jñānaṁ jñāninas tattva-darśinaḥ

One should approach a guru to learn about *tattva,* the Absolute Truth, not to acquire some material benefit. One should not search out a guru to cure some material disease. For that there is a medical practitioner. Why should you search out a guru for that purpose? A guru is one who knows the Vedic *śāstras,* or scriptures, and who can teach us to understand Kṛṣṇa.

Of course, we cannot understand Kṛṣṇa fully. That is not possible. We have no such capacity, because Kṛṣṇa is so great and we are so limited. Kṛṣṇa is so great that even He does not understand Himself. He does not know why He is so attractive. Therefore, to understand what makes Him so attractive He came as Lord Caitanya, adopting the ecstatic emotions of Śrīmatī Rādhārāṇī. So to understand Kṛṣṇa fully is not possible, but if we try to understand Him as far as our limited capacity allows, that is our perfection. That is why Kṛṣṇa says,

janma karma ca me divyam evaṁ yo vetti tattvataḥ
tyaktvā dehaṁ punar janma naiti mām eti so 'rjuna

"One who knows the transcendental nature of My appearance and activities does not, upon leaving the body, take his birth again in this material world, but attains My eternal abode, O Arjuna" [*Bhagavad-gītā* 4.9].

If we think that Kṛṣṇa is a human being like us, then we are *mūḍhas,* fools and rascals. We will be mistaken if we think, "Since my body is made of material elements, Kṛṣṇa's body is also made of material elements." In the *Bhagavad-gītā* Kṛṣṇa says that the material energy belongs to Him: *daivī hy eṣā guṇamayī mama māyā*. This material world is Kṛṣṇa's. We cannot say *mama māyā,* "This material energy is mine." No. We are under the control of the material nature. But Kṛṣṇa is the controller of the material nature: *mayādhyakṣeṇa prakṛtiḥ sūyate sa-carācaram*. That is the difference between Kṛṣṇa and us. Understanding that this material nature is working under the direction of Kṛṣṇa is real knowledge.

It is not possible to understand in detail how things are going on, but we can understand the summary: *janmādy asya yataḥ*. "Everything has emanated from the Supreme Absolute Truth, Kṛṣṇa." That much knowledge is sufficient. Then you can increase your knowledge—how the material nature is working under the direction of Kṛṣṇa, how Kṛṣṇa's energies are interacting, and so on. That is advanced knowledge. But if we simply understand Kṛṣṇa's statement in the *Bhagavad-gītā—mayādhyakṣeṇa prakṛtiḥ sūyate sa-carācaram:* "This material energy is working under my direction"—that is perfect knowledge.

The modern scientists think that matter is working independently, that everything has evolved due to chemical evolution. No. Chemical evolution cannot produce life. Life comes from life. As Kṛṣṇa says in the *Bhagavad-gītā, ahaṁ sarvasya prabhavo mattaḥ sarvaṁ pravartate:* "Everything emanates from Me." This is the reply to the scientists. And the *Vedānta-sūtra* confirms, *athāto brahma-jijñāsā, janmādy asya yataḥ:* "Now one should inquire into the Supreme Brahman, which is that from whom everything emanates." The Supreme Brahman is Kṛṣṇa.

The whole world is a combination of two things: *jaḍa* and *cetana,* dull matter and living entities. Both come from Kṛṣṇa. As He says in the *Bhagavad-gītā,*

apareyam itas tv anyāṁ prakṛtiṁ viddhi me parām
jīva-bhūtāṁ mahā-bāho yayedaṁ dhāryate jagat

"Besides the inferior, material energy, there is My superior, spiritual energy, the living entities who are exploiting the material nature" [*Bhagavad-gītā* 7.5]. Why is the spiritual energy superior? Because the living entities are utilizing the material nature. For example, we advanced living entities, human beings, have created the modern civilization by utilizing matter. That is our superiority. In this way we have to acquire *tattva-jñāna,* understanding of the Absolute Truth.

The *Vedānta-sūtra* confirms that human life is meant for understanding the Absolute Truth: *athāto brahma-jijñāsā.* And the explanation of the *Vedānta-sūtra* is the *Śrīmad-Bhāgavatam.* The *Vedānta-sūtra* states that the Absolute Truth is *janmādy asya,* that from whom, or from which, everything has emanated. Now, what is the nature of that source? This question is answered in the *Śrīmad-Bhāgavatam: janmādy asya yataḥ anvayād itaratas ca artheṣu abhijñaḥ.* That source is *abhijñaḥ,* cognizant. Now, matter is not cognizant, so that source must be life. Therefore the modern scientific theory that life comes from matter is wrong. Life comes from life. And the *Śrīmad-Bhāgavatam* continues, *tene brahma hṛdā ya ādi-kavaye:* "He imparted the Vedic knowledge unto Lord Brahmā." So unless one is a living entity, how can he impart knowledge?

The *Śrīmad-Bhāgavatam* is the natural explanation of the *Vedānta-sūtra* by the same author, Vyāsadeva. In the verse under discussion it is said Vidura was *dvaipāyana-sakha,* a friend of Dvaipāyana. *Dvaipāyana* means Vyāsadeva. Vyāsadeva compiled the *Vedānta-sūtra* and then explained it in the *Śrīmad-Bhāgavatam* (*artho 'yaṁ brahma-sūtrāṇāṁ*). If we read some artificial commentary on the *Vedānta-sūtra,* we'll misunderstand. Generally, the Māyāvādīs [impersonalists] give prominence to the commentary by Śaṅkarācārya, called the *Śārīraka-bhāṣya.* But that commentary is unnatural. The natural commentary is by the author himself, Vyāsadeva.

According to our Vedic system, the *ācārya* [spiritual master] must understand the *Vedānta-sūtra* and explain it. Then he'll be accepted as an *ācārya.* Therefore both of the main *sampradāyas* [spiritual communities], the Māyāvādī *sampradāya* and the Vaiṣṇava *sampradāya*, have explained the *Vedānta-sūtra.* Otherwise, they would not have been recognized as authoritative. Without understanding the *Vedānta-sūtra,* nobody can understand what is Brahman, the Absolute Truth. Similarly, here it is said that Vidura understood transcendental knowledge (*ānvīkṣikyām*) from Maitreya. Who is Maitreya? *Dvaipāyana-sakha*, the friend of Vyāsadeva. One friend knows the other friend—what his position is, what his knowledge is. So since Maitreya was the friend of Vyāsadeva, that means he knows what Vyāsadeva knows.

So we have to approach a spiritual master who is in the disciplic succession of Vyāsadeva. Many people claim, "Oh, we are also following Vyāsadeva." But that following cannot be superficial. One has to actually follow Vyāsadeva. For example, Vyāsadeva accepted Kṛṣṇa as the Supreme Personality of Godhead. This is stated in the *Bhagavad-gītā,* in the section where Arjuna says to Kṛṣṇa, *paraṁ brahma paraṁ dhāma pavitraṁ paramaṁ bhavān:* "O Kṛṣṇa, you are Parabrahman, the Supreme Person." But one may say it was because Arjuna was the friend of Kṛṣṇa that he accepted Him as the Supreme. No. Arjuna gave evidence: "Vyāsadeva also accepts You as the Supreme Lord." Similarly, Vyāsadeva begins the *Śrīmad-Bhāgavatam,* his commentary on the *Vedānta-sūtra,* by saying *oṁ namo bhagavate vāsudevāya:* "I offer my obeisances unto Vāsudeva, Kṛṣṇa, the Supreme Personality of Godhead."

So if we actually are interested in understanding spiritual knowledge, we must approach an *ācārya,* and an *ācārya* is one who follows Vyāsadeva. In the verse under discussion, Maitreya, the friend of Vyāsadeva, is the *ācārya.* He is so exalted that he has been described as Bhagavān. In general, the word *bhagavān* indicates Kṛṣṇa, the Supreme Personality of Godhead (*kṛṣṇas tu bhagavān svayam*). But sometimes other powerful persons, such as Lord Brahmā, Lord Śiva, Nārada, Vyāsadeva, or Maitreya, are also addressed as Bhagavān. Although the actual Bhagavān is Kṛṣṇa, such persons are sometimes called Bhagavān because they have attained as much knowledge of Kṛṣṇa as possible. It is not possible to have cent percent knowledge of Kṛṣṇa. Nobody can have that. Even Brahmā and Śiva cannot have that. But those who follow Kṛṣṇa's instructions fully are also sometimes called Bhagavān. However, that Bhagavān is not an artificial Bhagavān. A real Bhagavān must know what Kṛṣṇa has taught and follow His instructions.

So, here it is said, *viduraṁ prīta,* "Vidura pleased Maitreya." Their conversation wasn't simply talking between friends. No. Vidura was eager to receive transcendental knowledge, and Maitreya was pleased with him. How can one please the spiritual master? That we have mentioned before: *praṇipātena paripraśnena sevayā.* You can please the guru simply by surrendering to him, inquiring from him, and by rendering him service: "Sir, I am your most obedient servant. Please accept me and give me instruction." Arjuna also followed this process. At the beginning of the *Bhagavad-gītā* He said to Kṛṣṇa, *śiṣyas te 'haṁ śādhi māṁ tvāṁ prapannam:* "I am Your disciple and a soul surrendered unto You. Please instruct me." Even though Arjuna was a very intimate friend of Kṛṣṇa, still, while learning the *Bhagavad-gītā* from Him he surrendered to Kṛṣṇa and said, "I am no longer your friend; I am your disciple. Now I am under Your full control. Please instruct me."

So this is the process of approaching a guru. You must be very inquisitive and ask questions, but not to challenge the spiritual master. It is said, *jijñāsuḥ śreya uttamam:* You should approach the spiritual master to understand the spiritual science. You shouldn't try to defeat him. One should not say, "I know better than you. Let us talk." No. That is not the proper way to approach a guru. You must find a guru to whom you can surrender (*praṇipātena*). If you cannot surrender to the guru, then don't waste your time and his time. First of all surrender to the bona fide guru. This is the process of understanding transcendental knowledge.

Thank you very much. Hare Kṛṣṇa.

The Shelter from All Dangers

In this talk Śrīla Prabhupāda declares, "Everyone has to understand the goal of life, why there is a struggle for existence, and whether there is any remedy, a process whereby we can live very peacefully, without any disturbances. These are the things to be learned in human life, and one should approach a bona fide spiritual master to learn them." (July 1976, Washington, D.C.)

'sādhya'-'sādhana'-tattva puchite nā jāni
kṛpā kari' saba tattva kaha ta' āpani"

[Sanātana Gosvāmī said to Lord Caitanya:] "Actually, I do not know how to inquire about the goal of life and the process for obtaining it. Please be merciful to me and explain all these truths" (*Caitanya-caritāmṛta, Madhya-līlā* 20.103).

Human life is meant for understanding *tattva,* the Absolute Truth. That is the special advantage of human life. But if a human being is not trained to inquire about the Absolute Truth, he is at a great disadvantage.

In human life there is a chance to make a solution to the whole problem—the struggle for existence, for the survival of the fittest. This struggle is going on life after life. But now, in human life, one can end that struggle by understanding the goal of life and being trained in how to achieve it. If that opportunity is refused to human society by the guardians, by the government, it is a great disservice.

Human beings should not be kept in the darkness of animal propensities. How many plants and creepers there are! How many animals! How many aquatics! We have come through all these species after many millions of years of evolution. And now we have a chance to escape from this painful process. Therefore the human being is advised to try to understand the goal of life: *tamasi mā jyotir gama*. "Don't stay in darkness. Go to the light." That is the Vedic injunction.

So, from the very beginning of life, children should be trained to inquire about the goal of life. But if they are kept in darkness, simply taught to eat, drink, be merry, and enjoy—that is not civilization. They must be given the opportunity to inquire more and more about the goal of life. What is the goal of life? To revive our intimate relationship with God.

As Caitanya Mahāprabhu explains, we are intimately related to God, but somehow we have fallen into this material world, and we are mistakenly accepting this body as our self. We are being trained only to see to our bodily interests, just like cats and dogs. The animals are interested in the body only. They have no other interest. But if a human being is kept in the same darkness, simply concerned with his body, that is a great disadvantage.

Sanātana Gosvāmī understood that, and therefore he asked Śrī Caitanya Mahāprabhu,

'ke āmi', 'kene āmāya jāre tāpa-traya'
ihā nāhi jāni——'kemane hita haya'

"Who am I? Why should there be such a struggle for existence? Why not an easy life, a peaceful life? Why do some elements give us opposition? I want to be happy, but there is opposition. Why?"

Even with a fly we have to fight. I am sitting, not doing any harm to the fly, but it attacks me and bothers me. Or you may be walking on the street, committing no offense, but from a house a dog begins to bark, "Why are you coming here? Why are you coming here?" There is no cause for his barking, but because he is a dog his business is to bark, "Why are you coming? Why are you coming?"

Similarly, the immigration department restricts our freedom to go from one place to another. The immigration official barks, "Why are you coming? Why are you coming?" In many places we have been refused entry—"No, you cannot enter. Go back."—and I had to go back.

So, in this material world you cannot live peacefully. Not at all. There are so many impediments. The scripture says, *padaṁ padaṁ yad vipadām:* "At every step there is danger." Danger not only from the lower animals but also from human society. No, our life is not very happy in this material world.

Therefore we should be advanced in inquiring, Why are there so many impediments? How can I become happy? What is the goal of my life? Asking these questions is human life, and Sanātana Gosvāmī is representing us in asking these questions of Śrī Caitanya Mahāprabhu.

By the mercy of Caitanya Mahāprabhu, or by the mercy of His servants, one can be enlightened as to what is the goal of life, why there is a struggle for existence, why there is death, why there is birth. I do not want to die, I do not want to enter into a mother's womb and remain in a packed-up condition for so many days, I do not want to become an old man—but these things are forced upon me. Why? Our real business is to answer this question, not to arrange for economic development.

Whatever economic development we are destined to get, we shall get it. Whatever happiness or distress we are destined to get, we shall get it. We don't try for distress, but it comes; it is forced upon us. Similarly, although you don't try for it, the little happiness you are destined to obtain will also come. Therefore the scripture advises, "Instead of wasting your time bothering about so-called happiness and distress, better to engage your valuable time in understanding what is the goal of life, why there are so many problems, why you have to struggle for existence. This is your business."

In this Kṛṣṇa consciousness movement we are giving people a chance to understand the problems of life and how to solve them. It is not a sectarian movement or a so-called religious movement. It is not a religion. It is an educational and cultural movement. Everyone has to understand the goal of life, why there is a struggle for existence, and whether there is any remedy, a process whereby we can live very peacefully, without any disturbances. These are the things to be learned in human life, and one should approach a bona fide spiritual master to learn them.

This is what Sanātana Gosvāmī did. He was a government minister, very educated and well placed, but he approached Caitanya Mahāprabhu and humbly surrendered. So we should also approach Lord Caitanya or His representative and surrender (*tad viddhi praṇipātena*). One shouldn't challenge, "Can you show me God?" No, this is not the way to approach the spiritual master. God is everywhere, but now you do not have the eyes to see Him. So this challenging attitude will not help us. We must be submissive. As Kṛṣṇa says in the *Bhagavad-gītā*, *tad viddhi praṇipātena paripraśnena sevayā:* "To understand the transcendental science, approach a spiritual master and humbly surrender to him, inquire from him, and serve him." Sanātana Gosvāmī is a perfect example. He is submitting himself very humbly before Śrī Caitanya Mahāprabhu.

So, first of all surrender (*praṇipātena*); then ask questions (*paripraśnena*). Don't waste your time questioning the spiritual master unless you are surrendered. You must be ready to accept the answers he gives. Then you may make an inquiry. If you think, "I have to test his answers because I am more learned and more advanced then he," then don't go to the spiritual master. First of all settle up in your mind that whatever answers the spiritual master gives, you'll accept. Then you can make an inquiry.

Sanātana Gosvāmī completely surrendered to Caitanya Mahāprabhu. Sanātana said, "Actually, I do not know how to inquire from You. So kindly tell me what the subject matter of inquiry should be and what the answers to such inquiry are. I am a completely blank slate; I am simply submitting myself to You." Sanātana was inquisitive about *sādhya,* the goal of life, and *sādhana,* the process by which one can attain the goal. But he said, "I do not know anything about these things, so I am simply depending on Your mercy." That is surrender.

In this way we can make advancement in our spiritual education. But we must also carry out the orders of the spiritual master. As Narottama Dāsa Ṭhākura says, *guru-mukha-*

padma-vākya cittete kariyā aikya: "Make the orders of the spiritual master your life and soul." And then, *āra nā kariha mane āśā:* "Do not think otherwise." Simply accept what he says.

Of course, first of all you must select who will be your spiritual master. You must know his qualifications. If you want to purchase gold, you must at least know where gold is available. If you are so foolish that you go to a butcher shop to buy diamonds or gold, then you'll be cheated. Similarly, if out of ignorance you approach the wrong person for spiritual guidance, you'll be cheated.

So, finding a bona fide guru requires intelligence and sincerity. If you are serious about understanding the goal of life, spiritual knowledge, then Kṛṣṇa will help you. He is situated in everyone's heart, and he understands when you are sincerely seeking the Absolute Truth. Then He gives direction: "Go to this person." Kṛṣṇa is already giving direction in every respect. We want to do so many things, and Kṛṣṇa is giving us the facility. As He says in the *Bhagavad-gītā* [18.61], *īśvaraḥ sarva-bhūtānāṁ hṛd-deśe 'rjuna tiṣṭhati bhrāmayan sarva-bhūtāni.* As the Supersoul in the heart, Kṛṣṇa is giving facilities to all living entities in their wanderings throughout the various species. But when one becomes very eager to understand Kṛṣṇa, or God, He is glad to give instruction: "Go to such-and-such person and submissively inquire from him. You'll be enlightened." *Guru-kṛṣṇa-prasāde pāya bhakti-latā-bīja:* By the mercy of the spiritual master and Kṛṣṇa one can make spiritual advancement. One must simply be sincere.

Thank you very much. Hare Kṛṣṇa.

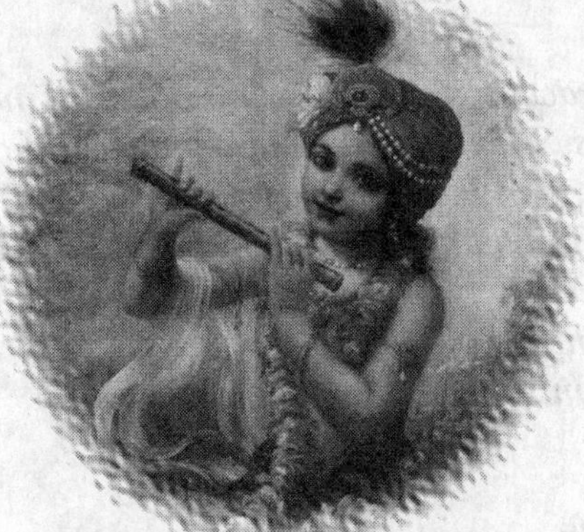

4.

Yoga and Meditation For the Age of Quarrel

Put Kṛṣṇa in the Center

It's easy to practice yoga when your object of meditation is all-attractive. As Śrīla Prabhupāda explains, "God is attractive for everyone, and God is equal to everyone. There is no distinction for God that here is an animal, here is a man, here is a tree. No. Every living entity is part and parcel of God. That is our understanding of God consciousness, or Kṛṣṇa consciousness." (September 1973, Stockholm, Sweden)

śrī-bhagavān uvāca
mayy āsakta-manāḥ pārtha yogaṁ yuñjan mad-āśrayaḥ
asaṁśayaṁ samagraṁ māṁ yathā jñāsyasi tac chṛṇu

"The Supreme Personality of Godhead said: 'Now hear, O son of Pṛthā [Arjuna], how by practicing yoga in full consciousness of Me, with mind attached to Me, you can know Me in full, free from doubt'" [*Bhagavad-gītā* 7.1].

This is a verse from the Seventh Chapter of the *Bhagavad-gītā,* which we have published as *Bhagavad-gītā As It Is*. There are many editions of the *Bhagavad-gītā,* and most of them have been edited to push forward the editor's own philosophical views. But we do not accept the *Bhagavad-gītā* in that light. The *Bhagavad-gītā* is spoken by the Supreme Personality of Godhead. It is stated here, *śrī bhagavān uvāca.* Those who are Sanskrit scholars will understand what is meant by the word *bhagavān*. *Bhaga* means "opulence," and one who possesses something is called *vān*. So *bhagavān* means "one who possesses all opulence."

There are six kinds of opulence: wealth, reputation, strength, beauty, knowledge, and renunciation. If a person is very rich, he attracts the attention of many persons. Similarly, if a man is very famous for his activities, he also attracts attention. If a person is very influential or strong, he also attracts attention. If a man or woman is very beautiful, he or she also attracts attention. And if one is very learned or renounced, he also attracts attention.

We all possess these opulences in some small quantity. Every one of us may possess some riches, may be a little wise or a little strong. But when you find that person who possesses more opulences than anyone else, that is God. The Sanskrit word for this is *asamordhva*. *Sama* means "equal," and *asama* means "not equal." And *ūrdhva* means "above." No one is equal to or greater than God. That is the definition of God. "God is great" means that nobody is equal to Him and nobody is above Him in any kind of opulence. That is called *bhagavān*.

Vyāsadeva writes *bhagavān* in the *Bhagavad-gītā* to describe Kṛṣṇa. The *Bhagavad-gītā* is one of the chapters of the *Mahābhārata*. The *Mahābhārata* means "the history of greater India." India is the name given by Westerners. But the real name is Bhārata-varṣa. Bhārata-varṣa means not only India but the whole planet. Five thousand years ago it was known as Bhārata-varṣa. Now the name Bhārata-varṣa indicates only India.

So the background of this *Bhagavad-gītā* is that there was a worldwide fight called the Battle of Kurukṣetra. Kurukṣetra is a place that still exists, and there was a battle there five thousand years ago. The main parties in the fight were cousin-brothers, the Kurus and the Pāṇḍavas. The *Bhagavad-gītā* was spoken there by Kṛṣṇa, the Supreme Personality of Godhead, Bhagavān.

Therefore, it is said *śrī bhagavān uvāca*. Kṛṣṇa is teaching Arjuna *bhakti-yoga*. Yoga is the means by which you can contact the Supreme. Yoga means "linking." There are many yoga systems for linking ourselves with the Supreme Absolute Truth.

The Absolute Truth is realized in three phases: impersonal, localized, and personal. In the *Śrīmad-Bhāgavatam* it is said that the Absolute Truth is realized by different persons according to different angles of vision. For example, if you see a mountain from a distant place, you see something cloudy. If you go nearer, then you find it is something green. And if you actually reach the mountain, then you find so many varieties. There are trees, there are houses, there are living entities, animals, everything. The object is one, but according to the vision of the person from the different distances, the same object is realized in different phases.

Therefore, the *Śrīmad-Bhāgavatam* says, *vadanti tat tattva-vidas tattvaṁ yaj jñānam advayam/brahmeti paramātmeti bhagavān iti śabdyate.* The object is one, but according to different understandings, somebody is realizing the Absolute Truth as impersonal Brahman, somebody is realizing the Absolute Truth as localized Paramātmā, and somebody is realizing the same Absolute Truth as the Supreme Personality of Godhead. Ultimately, the Absolute Truth is the Supreme Personality of Godhead, Bhagavān.

Therefore, Vyāsadeva, the compiler of the *Mahābhārata,* says, *śrī bhagavān uvāca.* So in this Kṛṣṇa consciousness movement we understand that Bhagavān is Kṛṣṇa. He has many millions of names, but Kṛṣṇa is the chief name. Kṛṣṇa means "the all-attractive." God must be all-attractive. It is not that God is attractive for one person and not for another. No. God is attractive for all living entities. Therefore, in pictures of Kṛṣṇa you see that He is loving the calves and cows, He is loving the trees, He is loving the *gopīs,* He is loving the cowherd boys. For Him, for God, everyone is a lovable object because everyone is the son of God.

Kṛṣṇa states in the *Bhagavad-gītā* that of the different species of life and different forms of life, "their mother is the material nature, and I am the seed-giving father."

God is attractive for everyone, and God is equal to everyone. There is no distinction for God that here is an animal, here is a man, here is a tree. No. Every living entity is part and parcel of God. That is our understanding of God consciousness, or Kṛṣṇa consciousness.

Among the different processes of yoga for linking to God, three are principal: *jñāna-yoga, dhyāna-yoga,* and *bhakti-yoga. Bhakti-yoga* is the topmost. That is described in the *Bhagavad-gītā* [6.47]:

yoginām api sarveṣāṁ mad-gatenāntar-ātmanā
śraddhāvān bhajate yo māṁ sa me yuktatamo mataḥ

Of all yogis, the yogi who is always thinking of Kṛṣṇa with love and faith is the first-class yogi.

The Seventh Chapter of the *Bhagavad-gītā* describes how to become a first-class yogi. Kṛṣṇa Himself explains how it is to be done. If you want to understand God, it is better to understand from God Himself. Instead of speculating about God, it is better to understand God from the words of God.

Vyāsadeva is the compiler of all Vedic knowledge, and he accepts Kṛṣṇa as the Supreme Personality of Godhead. Later on, all the *ācāryas*—Rāmānujācārya, Madhvācārya, Viṣṇu Svāmī, Lord Caitanya—they all accepted Kṛṣṇa. As far as our Vedic culture is concerned, Kṛṣṇa is the Supreme Personality of Godhead. Here it is also said, *śrī bhagavān uvāca*. Kṛṣṇa is teaching how to become a first-class yogi in Kṛṣṇa consciousness. He says, *mayy āsakta-manāḥ pārtha yogaṁ yuñjan mad-āśrayaḥ*. *Mayi* means "unto Me," and *āsakta* means "attachment." So He is saying that to become a first-class yogi one must increase his attachment to Kṛṣṇa.

The Kṛṣṇa consciousness yoga means to increase attachment for Kṛṣṇa. That's all. Everyone has attachment for something, either for his family or for some friend or for some house or some hobby or some cats, some dogs. There is attachment. That doesn't have to be learned. Attachment is there in everyone's heart. Everyone wants to be attached to somebody else; everyone wants to love someone else. Love does not mean oneness. For love there must be two: the lover and the beloved.

The Kṛṣṇa consciousness yoga system is the means to increase your attachment for Kṛṣṇa. Therefore it is said here, *mayy āsakta-manāḥ pārtha*—"gradually increasing one's attachment for Me." Kṛṣṇa says one should practice this yoga system by taking shelter of Him. You can take shelter directly of Kṛṣṇa, or you can take shelter of a person who has taken shelter of Kṛṣṇa. That is the meaning of *mad-āśraya*. That is the system of *paramparā,* disciple succession. Whether you increase your attachment for Kṛṣṇa or for a devotee of Kṛṣṇa, it is the same.

For example, if something is charged with electricity and you touch something else to it, it also becomes electrified. We have daily experience. The wires distribute the electricity from the powerhouse, and as soon as we join the plug, immediately it is electrified. Similarly, if you carry the words of Kṛṣṇa as they are carried by others in the disciplic succession, then you are in touch with Kṛṣṇa. That is called *yogaṁ yuñjan mad-āśrayaḥ:* always being linked with Kṛṣṇa.

Kṛṣṇa says in this verse, "Please try to hear from Me." Kṛṣṇa is speaking personally. So if we accept the *Bhagavad-gītā* as it is, as instructed by Kṛṣṇa Himself, then we can understand God without any doubt.

In our present position, with blunt material senses, with four defects, it is not possible to understand what God is. We have four defects in this material condition: we commit mistakes, we are illusioned, we tend to cheat, and our senses are imperfect. Every day we see the sun with our eyes, but because our senses are imperfect we see the sun as a disk, although it is thousands of times bigger than the earth. In this way, if we analyze our senses we will find that they are imperfect. Speculation based on imperfect senses is also imperfect. Therefore all the speculators—so-called scientists, philosophers, and so on—put forward theories: "Perhaps." "It may be." That means they do not have perfect knowledge. But if you receive knowledge from the supreme perfect, God, that is actually perfect.

Our process is like that. In the Fourth Chapter of the *Bhagavad-gītā,* Kṛṣṇa says He spoke this philosophy of the *Bhagavad-gītā* first to the sun-god, who spoke it to his son Manu, who spoke to his son Ikṣvāku. In this way, by disciple succession, the *Bhagavad-gītā* has come down to this earth. If we accept that disciplic succession instead of unnecessarily interpreting Kṛṣṇa's words, then we can understand the *Bhagavad-gītā*. That is the process.

Our Kṛṣṇa consciousness movement gives an understanding of the Supreme Personality of Godhead, Kṛṣṇa, as He is, without any interpretation. That is Kṛṣṇa consciousness yoga. That can be achieved, as Kṛṣṇa says, by always keeping Him in the center. If you practice this yoga, keeping Kṛṣṇa in the center and always thinking of the form of Kṛṣṇa, then Kṛṣṇa will be revealed to you. This is the yoga system of Kṛṣṇa consciousness.

Thank you very much.

Reaching Kṛṣṇa His Way

There are many paths, and they all don't *lead to the same goal. As Śrīla Prabhupāda says, "One has to come to the point of Kṛṣṇa consciousness. You may follow the yoga process, you may follow the philosophical process, you may follow the ritualistic process, or you may perform penances or engage in studying the Vedas. But unless you reach the point of Kṛṣṇa consciousness, you will succeed only to a certain degree." (November 1966, New York)*

na sādhayati māṁ yogo na sāṅkhyaṁ dharma uddhava
na svādhyāyas tapas tyāgo yathā bhaktir mamorjitā

[The Supreme Personality of Godhead, Kṛṣṇa, said:] "My dear Uddhava, neither through *aṣṭāṅga-yoga* [the mystic yoga system to control the senses], nor through impersonal monism or an analytical study of the Absolute Truth, nor through study of the *Vedas,* nor through austerities, charity, or acceptance of *sannyāsa* can one satisfy Me as much as by developing unalloyed devotional service unto Me" [*Śrīmad-Bhāgavatam* 11.14.20].

Lord Caitanya quoted this verse while relating an allegory in which an astrologer tells a poor man where to dig to find a treasure. The treasure represents Kṛṣṇa consciousness, or love of God, and the directions in which the man is told to dig represent different processes by which people search for the Absolute Truth.

The astrologer tells the poverty-stricken man, "You are actually a very rich man's son, but you do not know this. Therefore you are suffering."

To be poor in this world is a curse for ordinary people, those under the concept of material life, whereas the spiritually enriched have nothing to do with the poverty or wealth of this world. The living entities are not meant to be poverty-stricken, because they are part and parcel of the Supreme

Lord, the supreme proprietor. Every living entity has the birthright to enjoy God's property, just as the son inherits the property of the father. That is the law. But under the spell of illusion we have forgotten our relationship with the supreme father; therefore we are suffering. That is the diagnosis.

Now we have to find out how to go back home, back to Godhead. That should be the mission of human life. Never mind why we are in contact with the material world. By the instruction of the astrologerlike Vedic literature we should come to the point of finding out how to go back to Godhead. Just as the astrologer is giving hints to the poor man, the Vedic literature gives us hints so that we can become the richest by reviving our lost relationship with our father.

There are different paths for reviving that relationship, but Lord Caitanya says that no method but *bhakti* will work. The Vedic literature says the same thing. In the verse under discussion Lord Caitanya is citing evidence from the *Śrīmad-Bhāgavatam,* where Lord Kṛṣṇa is instructing his cousin-brother Uddhava just as He instructed Arjuna in the *Bhagavad-gītā*. Kṛṣṇa says, *na sādhayati māṁ yogaḥ:* "By adopting the yoga process one cannot succeed in reaching Me." And then, *na sāṅkhyaṁ dharma uddhava:* "Nor will philosophical speculation or ordinary religious principles help one reach Me, O Uddhava."

Real yoga means "connect, plus, addition." In mathematics we have addition and subtraction. So at the present moment we are in subtraction—God minus myself. I have no sense of God; therefore I am in a "minus" condition. Yoga means God plus myself. That is the real meaning of yoga. For so long I was God-minus; now, through yoga, I become God-plus.

But you must always remember that in the spiritual, absolute sense God plus me is God and God minus me is also God. When I am "minus," or separated from God, that does not mean God has lost some of His capacity. No. He is full. And when I am "plus," or reunited with God, that does not mean God has increased in some capacity. No.

In the *Bhagavad-gītā* Kṛṣṇa gives a good example: *āpūryamāṇam acala-pratiṣṭhaṁ samudram*. During the rainy season millions of tons of water pour into the ocean from rivers, but the ocean stays the same. If an ordinary ocean does not increase when something is added to it, what to speak of God?

I say "ordinary" because millions of oceans are floating in the universe. Therefore we should not be very astonished to see the Atlantic Ocean. Within space are millions and trillions of oceans like the Atlantic. They are floating just as an atomic particle of water can float in the air. That is the potency of God.

For those who are too engrossed in the bodily conception of life, the yoga system is very good, because it is a practice to withdraw the senses from their engagement in the external world. There are eight stages of yoga practice. The first two are *yama* and *niyama*. Under regulative principles one has to try to control the senses in eating, sleeping, and working. That practice is called *yama-niyama*. The first principle of yoga is to abstain from sex life. That is real yoga. Those indulging in sex life, intoxication, and so many nonsense things have no chance for any success in yoga.

Then one has to sit nicely in a secluded, sanctified place with the neck, head, and body in a straight line. Then you have to look at the tip of your nose with half-opened eyes. If you open your eyes, then the material manifestation will disturb you. And if you close your eyes, then you nap. [*Śrīla Prabhupāda imitates someone snoring.*] I have seen it. So many "yogis" are doing that, sleeping. [*Laughter.*]

Another step in the eightfold yoga system is *dhāraṇā,* concentration of the mind. What is the purpose of concentrating the mind? To find my self within the body and then find the Lord there. That is the perfection of yoga. Not that I do nonsense day and night but then attend a yoga class, pay five dollars, and think, "Oh, I am a great yogi." That is all nonsense.

Yoga is not so easy. Many so-called yoga teachers are simply exploiting people. I say frankly that they and their students are a society of the cheaters and the cheated.

Although yoga is approved in the Vedic literature, it is very difficult to perform in the modern age. Even five thousand years ago—when the circumstances were more favorable, when people were not so polluted and were advanced in so many things—still, at that time such a person as Arjuna refused to practice yoga. When Kṛṣṇa said to him, "You become a yogi like this," Arjuna said, "It is not possible for me."

So yoga is not at all possible now. It was possible in the Satya-yuga, when every man was in the mode of goodness, every man was highly elevated. Yoga is meant for highly elevated persons, not ordinary persons.

But even if yoga is done very nicely and perfectly, it cannot take you to the Supreme Lord. That is stated here in this verse. What to speak of pseudo yoga, even if you perform yoga perfectly, still you cannot reach God. That is stated here: *na sādhayati māṁ yogaḥ.*

It is also said here, *na sāṅkhyaṁ:* "Not by Sāṅkhya." Sāṅkhya means to understand spirit and matter. Sāṅkhya philosophers describe the material world as made of twenty-four parts: the five gross elements, the three subtle elements, the five knowledge-acquiring senses, the five working senses, the five sense objects, and *pradhāna,* the unmanifested modes of material nature. The five gross material elements are earth, water, fire, air, and ether. Then come the subtle elements. Finer than ether is the mind, finer than the mind is the intelligence, and finer than the intelligence is false ego, the false conception that I am matter. The five knowledge-acquiring senses are the eyes, nose, ears, tongue, and skin. The five working senses are the voice, legs, hands, anus, and genitals. And the five sense objects are smell, taste, form, touch, and sound.

That analysis of the material world into twenty-four parts is called Sāṅkhya. It is a full analysis of everything within our experience. And above the twenty-four elements is the spirit soul. And above the soul is God.

Sāṅkhyites cannot find the soul. They are like material scientists in that they simply study material objects. They have no information above that. Now I am talking with you; so the Sāṅkhya philosophers cannot explain what is that thing which is talking. Similarly, the medical doctor, after dissecting the body, cannot find what is working, the spiritual force. And because the materialists cannot find even the particles of the Supreme Lord—us living entities—what chance do they have of finding God? So neither the yogis nor the Sāṅkhyites can find God.

By dharma, also, one cannot find God. Dharma here refers to rituals. The Hindus go to the temple, the Christians go to the church, and the Muslims go to the mosque with the idea "Here is God." That is, of course, the beginning. It is nice. That conviction must be there. But because they are trapped in the rituals, they have no further knowledge. They do not try to advance further. They think, "Everything ends here." So they too cannot attain God.

Then *svādhyāya. Svādhyāya* means "study," study of the Vedic literature. And *tapa. Tapa* means "penance." Fasting, meditating, living in a solitary place in the jungle—there are many processes of penance and austerity. And *tyāga,* "renunciation." *Sannyāsa,* the renounced order of life, is the emblem of renunciation.

So the Lord says, "All these processes—yoga, Sāṅkhya, rituals, study of the *Vedas,* penance, and renunciation—combined together or practiced individually, are not suitable for achieving Me."

So practically all processes are condemned herewith by the Supreme Lord. Condemned in this sense: those who follow them can approach the final goal to a certain extent, but they will never be able to achieve it unless the devotional process is added. Devotion must be there because the end is Kṛṣṇa, the Supreme Lord. Kṛṣṇa says in the *Bhagavad-gītā, bahūnāṁ janmanām ante jñānavān māṁ prapadyate:* "After many, many births, those who are actually intelligent come to Me and surrender, having realized that God is everything."

One has to come to the point of Kṛṣṇa consciousness. You

may follow the yoga process, you may follow the philosophical process, you may follow the ritualistic process, or you may perform penances or engage in studying the *Vedas*. But unless you reach the point of Kṛṣṇa consciousness, you will succeed only to a certain degree.

Unfortunately, people become satisfied with different degrees of success. Hardly anyone tries to reach the final goal. But if anyone wants to reach the final goal, then he has to take up the process of Kṛṣṇa consciousness (*bhaktir mamorjitā*). That process alone can take you to the Supreme Lord.

Those who are intelligent take to the simple process of Kṛṣṇa consciousness. In this age you cannot perform yoga perfectly, you cannot perform religious rituals perfectly, you cannot study perfectly. The circumstances are so unfavorable that these processes are not possible in this age. Therefore Lord Caitanya, by His causeless mercy, has given us the process of Kṛṣṇa consciousness, beginning with the chanting of the holy name. And His teaching is corroborated in the *Bṛhan-nāradīya Purāṇa*:

harer nāma harer nāma harer nāmaiva kevalam
kalau nāsty eva nāsty eva nāsty eva gatir anyathā

"In this Age of Kali, simply by chanting the holy name of Kṛṣṇa one can attain the ultimate goal. There is no alternative. There is no alternative. There is no alternative."

So Lord Caitanya has not manufactured something by recommending *bhakti* as the only means to the ultimate goal. He is quoting from authorized scripture so that people can accept the path of *bhakti*. Therefore we should accept this process, especially the chanting of the Hare Kṛṣṇa *mantra,* and if we follow it very seriously and sincerely we will practically see that this is the only process for swiftly realizing the Supreme Truth, the Absolute Truth.

Thank you very much.

How to See and Know God

In this talk Śrīla Prabhupāda sharply distinguishes between human beings and animals: "One's spiritual life begins when one asks, What am I? Why have I come here? Why am I put into so many miserable conditions? Is there any remedy? Human life is meant for answering these questions. . . . [But] if one is simply directed by the urges of the senses, one is no better than the ducks and dogs." (October 1968, Seattle, Washington)

We are worshiping Govinda, the Supreme Personality of Godhead, the original person. And this song we were just singing—*govindam ādi-puruṣaṁ tam ahaṁ bhajāmi*—is reaching Him. He's hearing it. You cannot say He's not hearing it. Especially in this scientific age, when radio messages are broadcast thousands and thousands of miles so you can hear them, it is easy to understand how Govinda, Kṛṣṇa, can hear your sincere prayer.

Similarly, just as you can see a television picture transmitted from thousands and thousands of miles away, you can always see Govinda in your heart if you prepare yourself properly. This is stated in the *Brahma-saṁhitā* [5.38]: *premāñjana-cchurita-bhakti-vilocanena santaḥ sadaiva hṛdayeṣu vilokayanti.* There is a television within your heart; it is not that you have to purchase the television set—it is there in your heart. And God is also there. You can see Him, you can hear Him, you can talk with Him, provided you repair the machine. And this repairing process is Kṛṣṇa consciousness.

Now, to repair a television an expert technician is required. Similarly, you require the help of someone expert in the science of Kṛṣṇa consciousness. Then the machine in your heart will work and you will be able to see Kṛṣṇa. This is the perfection of yoga.

In the scriptures we hear how one can come to this perfection: *sādhu-śāstra-guru-vākya, cittete kariyā aikya.* Spiritual realization can be perfected by following three parallel lines: *sādhu* (saintly persons who are realized souls), *śāstra* (authoritative Vedic scriptures), and *guru* (the spiritual master). In the railway yard you see two parallel tracks, and if they're in order the railway carriages go very smoothly to their destination. In Kṛṣṇa consciousness there are three parallel lines: association with saintly persons (*sādhus*), faith in the scriptures (*śāstra*), and acceptance of a bona fide spiritual master (*guru*). If you place your vehicle on these three parallel lines, it will go directly to Kṛṣṇa, without any disturbance.

Now, here in the *Bhagavad-gītā,* Kṛṣṇa, the Supreme Personality of Godhead, is explaining Himself. But suppose you say, "How can I believe that Kṛṣṇa said these words? Somebody may have written them in the name of Kṛṣṇa." No. Because the *Bhagavad-gītā* is accepted by saintly persons, we should also accept it. Beginning from Vyāsadeva and Nārada, down to many *ācāryas* [spiritual exemplars] like Rāmānujācārya, Madhvācārya, Viṣṇu Svāmī, and Lord Caitanya, all have accepted the *Bhagavad-gītā:* "Yes, it is spoken by God, Kṛṣṇa." So this is the proof that the *Bhagavad-gītā* is authentic. Saintly persons, *sādhus,* have accepted the *Bhagavad-gītā* as scripture; therefore it is scripture. That is the test.

This is a common-sense affair. If lawyers accept some book as a law book, then we should understand that it is an authoritative law book. You cannot say, "Why should I accept this law book?" The evidence is that the lawyers have accepted it. Similarly, if the medical practitioners accept a book as authoritative, then we should know that it is an authoritative medical book. In the same way, since saintly persons accept the *Bhagavad-gītā* as scripture, you cannot deny that it is scripture. So these are the two lines of *sādhu* and *śāstra,* saintly persons and scripture.

And who is a *guru,* a spiritual master? He who follows and explains the scripture. The *sādhu* confirms the scripture, and the spiritual master follows and explains the scripture. So *sādhu, śāstra,* and *guru* are always in agreement. What is spoken in the scripture is accepted by saintly persons, and what is spoken in the scripture is followed and explained by the spiritual master, and he explains *only* that. The via media is the scripture, just as in the law court the via media is the law book. So the saintly persons, the scriptures, and the spiritual master: when you follow these three parallel lines your life is successful.

Now, in the beginning of the Seventh Chapter of the *Bhagavad-gītā* Kṛṣṇa speaks about yoga. In the first six chapters He explains the constitutional position of the living entity. Until that is understood, your activities in yoga, in relation to Kṛṣṇa, cannot actually begin. Suppose you are working in an office. If your post is not settled up—if you don't know what duties you have to execute—you cannot do anything very nicely. The typist, the clerk, the errand boy—they are executing their work very nicely because they understand their duties. Therefore, to practice yoga one first has to understand the constitutional position of the living entity, and that is explained in the first six chapters of the *Bhagavad-gītā.*

So yoga means to understand one's constitutional position and to act in that position. The first step is controlling the senses (*yoga indriya-saṁyama*). Now everyone is busy gratifying the senses. When you stand on the street, you see that everybody is very busy. The storekeeper is busy, the motorcar driver is busy—everyone is very busy. How are they busy? If you minutely study their business, you will find that their only business is sense gratification. That's all. Everyone is busy trying to gratify his senses. This is material life. And spiritual life, or *yoga,* means to control the senses and understand our constitutional position as spirit souls.

One's spiritual life begins when one asks, What am I? Why have I come here? Why am I put into so many miserable conditions? Is there any remedy? Human life is meant for answering these questions. Animals do not know anything except sense gratification. They have no power of understanding; their consciousness is not developed. For example, in

Green Lake Park there are many ducks. As soon as somebody goes there with a little food, they gather: "*Kaa, kaa, kaa, kaa.*" And after eating, they enjoy sex. That's all. The life of cats and dogs is like that also, and human life is also like that if one never asks, What am I? If one is simply directed by the urges of the senses, one is no better than the ducks and dogs.

So in the first six chapters of the *Bhagavad-gītā* Kṛṣṇa explains that the living entity is a spiritual spark. It is very difficult to find out where the spark is because it is so minute. No microscope can find it out. But it is there in your body. Because it is in your body, you are moving, you are talking, you are planning—you are doing so many things simply by the influence of that spiritual spark.

We are very minute sparks of the supreme spirit, just like particles of sunshine. The sun's rays are made up of shining particles, and when these shining particles mix together they form sunshine. Similarly, we are minute particles of God, and because we are part and parcel of God we have the same propensities as God: thinking, feeling, willing, creating—everything. Whatever you see in yourself is there in God also. Therefore, since we are all persons, God cannot be impersonal. I have so many propensities in a very minute quantity, and the same propensities are there in Kṛṣṇa, or God, in an unlimited quantity. This is the science of Kṛṣṇa consciousness.

We are small, infinitesimal, yet we still have so many propensities, so many desires, so many activities, so much brainwork. Just imagine how much greater are God's desires and activities and brainwork! So qualitatively God and the living entity are one, but quantitatively we are different. He is great, we are small. He is infinite, we are infinitesimal.

Now, when sparks are in the fire they glow very nicely, but when they are out of the fire they are extinguished. Similarly, since we are sparks of Kṛṣṇa, when we associate with Him our illuminating quality is manifested. Otherwise, we are practically extinguished, or covered. The living spark cannot be extinguished. If it were extinguished, how are we manifesting our living condition? No, it is not extinguished; it is covered. When a fire is covered you can feel heat on the cover, but you cannot see the fire directly. Similarly, when the spiritual spark is covered by the material dress, the body, you can see the effects of the spark—your activities of life—but you cannot see the spark directly. To see the spiritual spark directly, to uncover your original spiritual nature, you must practice yoga.

In the first verse of the Sixth Chapter of the *Bhagavad-gītā,* Kṛṣṇa explains the *yoga* process: *mayy āsakta-manāḥ pārtha yogaṁ yuñjan mad-āśrayaḥ.* You have to constantly engage your mind in thoughts of Kṛṣṇa. That is the yoga process we are presenting as Kṛṣṇa consciousness. And it is not very difficult. Kṛṣṇa is beautiful, all-attractive, and He has many activities. The Vedic literature is full of Kṛṣṇa's activities. And the *Bhagavad-gītā* is full of Kṛṣṇa's teachings. Simply understanding that God is great is a neutral state of understanding. You have to elevate yourself more and more by understanding *how* great He is. Of course, it is not possible to fully understand how great He is, because our senses are always imperfect, but as far as possible we should try. You can hear about the activities of God, about the position of God, and you can put your argument and make your judgment. Then you will understand without any doubt what God is.

So real yoga is *mayy āsakta-manāḥ,* always thinking of Kṛṣṇa. At the end of the Sixth Chapter of the *Bhagavad-gītā* Kṛṣṇa explains that one who is constantly absorbed in thoughts of Him is a first-class yogi. In Western countries yoga has become very popular, but most people do not know who is a first-class yogi. Kṛṣṇa says, *yoginām api sarveṣāṁ mad-gatenāntarātmanā . . . sa me yuktatamo mataḥ:* "Out of many thousands of yogis, he who is always seeing the form of Kṛṣṇa within his heart is first class."

So you have to practice that first-class yoga system, which Kṛṣṇa describes as *mayy āsakta-manāḥ:* "Make your mind attached to Me." The mind is the vehicle for attachment, and generally we become attached to a person—a boy, a girl, and so on. Impersonal attachment is bogus. So yoga begins by attaching the mind to Kṛṣṇa by always thinking of Him, and it culminates in love of Kṛṣṇa. For example, there are many nice paintings of Śrīmatī Rādhārāṇī with Kṛṣṇa in Vṛndāvana. So you can always think of such a picture; then you will constantly be in *samādhi* [yogic trance]. Why try to think of something impersonal, some void? If you try to think of the void, you will start thinking of some light, some color—so many things will come into your mind. The mind *must* think of some form. How can we avoid form? It is not possible. Therefore, why not concentrate your mind on the supreme form, Kṛṣṇa?

Īśvaraḥ paramaḥ kṛṣṇaḥ sac-cid-ānanda-vigrahaḥ. The Supreme Personality of Godhead, the supreme controller, is Kṛṣṇa, and He has a body. What sort of body? *Sac-cid-ānanda:* an eternal body full of bliss and knowledge. Not a body like ours. Our body is full of ignorance, full of miseries, and not eternal—just the opposite of Kṛṣṇa's. His body is eternal, my body is not eternal. His body is full of bliss, my body is full of miseries. There is always something troubling us: headache, toothache, this ache, that ache. Somebody is giving us personal trouble, we are feeling severe heat, severe cold—so many things. But Kṛṣṇa's form, Kṛṣṇa's body, is eternally full of bliss and knowledge.

So Kṛṣṇa consciousness means always thinking of Kṛṣṇa's form, name, pastimes, and so on. How can we practice this yoga system, Kṛṣṇa consciousness? *Mayy āsakta-manāḥ pārtha yogaṁ yuñjan mad-āśrayaḥ. Mad-āśrayaḥ* means "taking shelter of somebody who is in touch with Me." As soon as you think of Kṛṣṇa you are in direct touch with Him. But unless you take shelter of a spiritual master who knows about Him, you cannot concentrate for a long time. Therefore, if you want to concentrate on Kṛṣṇa continuously, you have to hear from a person who knows about Kṛṣṇa, and you have to act according to his directions. Your life should be molded according to the directions of the spiritual master. Then you can practice yoga perfectly.

As mentioned before, Kṛṣṇa explains the perfection of yoga in the last verse of the Sixth Chapter of the *Bhagavad-gītā. Yoginām api sarveṣāṁ mad-gatenāntarātmanā . . . sa me yuktatamo mataḥ:* "One who is always thinking of Me is a first-class yogi." So we have to place Kṛṣṇa in our mind; we have to always think of Him. How? Kṛṣṇa explains [Bg. 7.1],

mayy āsakta-manāḥ pārtha yogaṁ yuñjan mad-āśrayaḥ
asaṁśayaṁ samagraṁ māṁ yathā jñāsyasi tac chṛṇu

"Under My protection, under the protection of My representative, always think of Me. Then you will understand Me perfectly well, without doubt, and your life will be successful." *Asaṁśayaṁ* means "without any doubt." If you doubt that Kṛṣṇa is the Supreme Personality of Godhead, just put forward your questions and try to understand. It is undoubtedly a fact that He is the Supreme Personality of Godhead, but if you have some doubt, you can clear it up by placing questions before the spiritual master.

So if you practice Kṛṣṇa consciousness, the topmost of all yoga systems, in this way, then without any doubt you'll understand Kṛṣṇa, the Supreme Personality of Godhead, perfectly well. And your life will be successful.

Thank you very much.

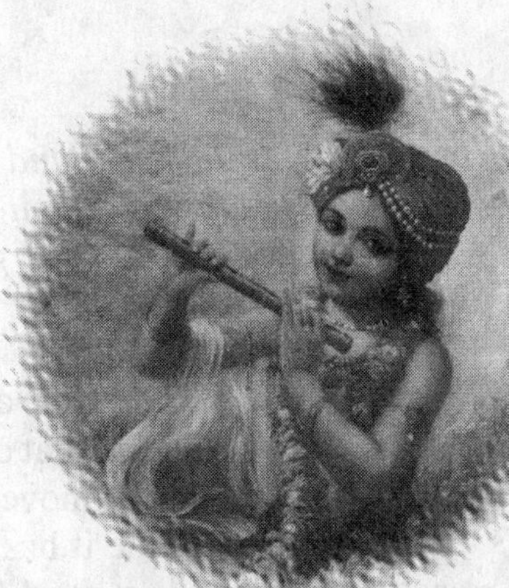

5.

Spiritual Solutions to Material Problems

Advice to the United Nations

How can society be organized for the peace and well-being of all? Śrīla Prabhupāda discusses this question with Mr. C. Hennis of the U.N.'s International Labor Organization in Geneva, Switzerland, in May of 1974.

Śrīla Prabhupāda: The social body should have a class of men who act as the brain and guide everyone so that everyone can become happy. That is the purpose of our movement.
Mr. Hennis: That's a valid point, because it has always been affirmed in every society that there is a need for a priestly class or a class of philosophical leaders.
Śrīla Prabhupāda: But now the so-called priestly class are amending the Biblical injunctions according to their whims. For instance, the Bible enjoins, "Thou shalt not kill." But the priestly class is like the other classes—sanctioning slaughterhouses. So how can they guide?
Mr. Hennis: But the animal world is entirely composed of beings who eat one another. I suppose that the justification that people have for maintaining slaughterhouses is that it is just a cleaner way of killing than for a lion to jump on the back of an antelope.
Śrīla Prabhupāda: But as a human being you should have discrimination. You should be guided by your brain, and society should be guided by the "brain class" of priestly, thoughtful men. Nature has given human beings the fruits, the vegetables, the grains, the milk, which all have great nutritional value, and human beings should be satisfied with these wholesome foods. Why should they maintain slaughterhouses? And how can they think they will be happy by being sinful, by disobeying God's commandments? This means society has no brain.
Mr. Hennis: My organization isn't directly concerned with giving people brains.
Śrīla Prabhupāda: Your organization may not be directly

concerned. But if human society is brainless, no matter how much you may try to organize, society can never be happy. That is my point.

Mr. Hennis: My organization is concerned with taking away the obstacles that prevent people from attaining a proper brain. One of the obstacles is just plain poverty.

Śrīla Prabhupāda: No. The main thing is, society must learn to discriminate between pious and sinful activities. Human beings must engage in pious activities, not sinful activities. Otherwise, they have no brain. They are no better than animals. And from the moral point of view, do you like sending your mother to the slaughterhouse? You are drinking the milk of the cow—so she is your mother—and after that you are sending her to the slaughterhouse. That is why we ask. Where is society's brain?

Mr. Hennis: Of course, when we speak of the distinctions that are made between pious activities and sinful activities—

Śrīla Prabhupāda: Today practically no one is making this distinction. We are making it, and we have introduced these ideas by establishing farm communities and protecting our cows. And our cows are winning awards for giving the most milk, because they are so jubilant. They know, "These people will not kill me." They know it, so they are very happy. Nor do we kill their calves. At other farms, soon after the cow gives birth to a calf, they pull her calf away for slaughter. You see? This means society has no brain. You may create hundreds of organizations, but society will never be happy. That is the verdict.

Mr. Hennis: Well, we can't be accused of engaging in sinful activities when we don't think what we are doing is sinful.

Śrīla Prabhupāda [*Laughing*]: Oh? You don't think you can be accused of breaking the state law—just because you don't know what the state law is? The point is, if your priestly class have no knowledge of what is sinful, they may instruct you, "Don't do anything sinful"—but what good is that? You must have a priestly class who know what is sinful, so that they can teach you. And then you must give up your sinful activities.

When these young people came to me, I told them, "Flesh-eating, illicit sex, gambling, and intoxication—these things are sinful. You must give them up." If we do not give up these sinful activities, nature punishes us. So we must know the laws of nature, what nature wants. At the very least, nature wants that we human beings stop our sinful activities. If we do not, then we must be punished.

Mr. Hennis: We are just trying to give people a fair share of the material things of life: proper wages, decent homes, decent opportunities for leisure.

Śrīla Prabhupāda: That is all right, but people must know what is sinful and what is pious.

Mr. Hennis: Yes, but I don't think you can properly expect to indoctrinate people. At least, you can't expect an international organization to indoctrinate people.

Śrīla Prabhupāda: As an international organization for peace and well-being, the United Nations should maintain a class of men who can act as society's brain. Then everything will be all right. Simply legs and hands working without any direction, without any brain—that is not very good. The United Nations was organized for the total benefit of human society, but it has no department that can actually be called the brain organization.

Mr. Hennis: That's true. That's true. They are servants of the membership, servants of the various states of the world. We are only servants of these people. What we try to do is let them get together and help them understand their problems.

Śrīla Prabhupāda: Yes, help them understand. At the very least, help them understand what they should do and what they should not do. At least do this much.

Mr. Hennis: This we do try to do to the extent that it is possible for the secretariat to shape and evolve a philosophy. We try to do it. But of course, we can't adopt a completely radical approach. We do what we can, in the manner of a good servant and the manner of a good steward, to try and hope the leaders are on the right path and the right direction.

Śrīla Prabhupāda: If society does not know what is sinful and what is pious, it is all useless. If your body has no brain, then your body is dead. And if the social body has no brain, then it is dead.

Back to Simple Life and Simple Truth

In this conversation with some of his disciples Śrīla Prabhupāda says, "Modern, artificial 'necessities of life' may seem to increase your so-called comfort. But if you forget life's real aim, your so-called advancement of technology is suicidal." (June 1976, the Hare Kṛṣṇa farming village at New Vrindaban, West Virginia)

Disciple: Śrīla Prabhupāda, once you said, "The tractor—this is the cause of all the trouble. It took all the young men's farm work. It forced them to go into the city and become entangled in sensuality." You said people had to leave the country and the simple life of goodness and God consciousness. And so they went to the city and got caught up in the anxious life, the mode of passion.

Śrīla Prabhupāda: Yes. In the city people must naturally fall into the mode of passion: constant anxiety due to needless lusting and striving. In the city we are surrounded by all sorts of artificial things for agitating our mind and senses. And naturally, when we have this facility we become lusty. We take to this passionate mode and become filled with anxiety.

Disciple: The country is more peaceful. It's easier to think of spiritual life.

Śrīla Prabhupāda: Yes. There is less disease. Everything is less brain-taxing. In the country the pangs of this material world are less. So you can arrange your life for real profit. Spiritual profit. Realize God; become Kṛṣṇa conscious. And if you have got a temple in your home or near your home, you have a very happy life. You work just a little—just for your food—in the spring a month and a half or so for planting, in the fall a month and a half for harvesting. And in your remaining time you become culturally and spiritually enriched. You engage all your talents and energies for realizing

God. Kṛṣṇa consciousness. This is ideal life.

You see the minute fibers on this flower? No other manufacturing process in this world can do this—such small fibers. And how brilliant is the color! If you study only one flower, you will become God conscious.

There is a mechanism that we call "nature." And from it is coming everything we see around us. Now, how is it that this mechanism is so perfect? And who is it that has devised this mechanism?

Disciple: Once in London you said, "People do not know that flowers are painted. Kṛṣṇa paints them with thoughts."

Śrīla Prabhupāda: Yes. Most people think that by itself, unconnected with a painter, this flower has become beautiful. This is foolishness. "Nature has done it." *Whose* nature? Everything is being done by the natural mechanism of Kṛṣṇa. *Parāsya śaktir vividhaiva śrūyate:* the Lord is orchestrating everything by His innumerable, inconceivable energies.

Anyway, learn to love this natural mode of life, life in a wide-open space. Produce your own grain. Produce your own milk. Save time. Chant Hare Kṛṣṇa. Glorify the Lord's holy names. At life's end, go back to the spiritual world to live forever. Plain living, high thinking—ideal life.

Modern, artificial "necessities of life" may seem to increase your so-called comfort, but if you forget life's real aim, your so-called advancement of technology is suicidal. We want to stop this suicidal policy.

People today are extremely attached to this so-called advancement. Therefore when Lord Caitanya appeared five hundred years ago, He gave a simple formula: chant Hare Kṛṣṇa. Even in your technological factory, you can chant. You go on pushing and pulling with your machine, and chant, "Hare Kṛṣṇa, Hare Kṛṣṇa." You can devote yourself to God. What is the wrong there?

Disciple: The leaders know that once a person starts chanting God's names, in time he'll lose his taste for this anxious life of technology.

Śrīla Prabhupāda: That is natural.

Disciple: So the leaders know you are sowing the seeds of their destruction.
Śrīla Prabhupāda: Where is the "destruction"? Rather, it is construction: devote yourself to God, and live forever. This is the proper path. Follow it. You will live forever.

By our method, *tyaktvā dehaṁ punar janma naiti:* after leaving your present material body, you don't get any more material bodies. You regain your spiritual body and go back to the spiritual world. And without this spiritual realization, *tathā dehāntara-prāptiḥ:* when you leave your present material body, you'll have to accept another material body.

So consider the two methods of living. Which is better? The "advanced" method—accepting more material bodies—or our "old-fashioned" method—accepting no more material bodies. Which is better?

As soon as you accept a material body, you have to suffer: birth, old age, disease, death. The material body means suffering. Therefore, if we prepare so that on leaving this present body we undergo no more suffering, that is intelligent. But if we prepare to receive another material body for more suffering, is that intelligent? Unless you understand the Lord, unless you understand Kṛṣṇa, you'll have to stay in this material world and accept another body. There is no alternative.

Now our method. We understand, first, that *na hanyate hanyamāne śarīre:* when the body is finished, the soul goes on living. Unfortunately, many people have become so dull-brained that they cannot understand this simple truth.

Every day of their lives people see that a soul in an infant body is going to take on a childhood body, then a teenage body, next an adult body, and later an aged body. People see, with their own eyes, how the soul is transmigrating from one body to another body to still another body.

Nevertheless, with their dull brains they cannot understand that at death, when the aged body is finished, the soul goes on to yet another body, material or spiritual. But people cannot understand this. They are so dull-brained. They cannot make the simple distinction between the body and the soul. It will take five hundred years to teach them this simple truth— their education is so advanced.

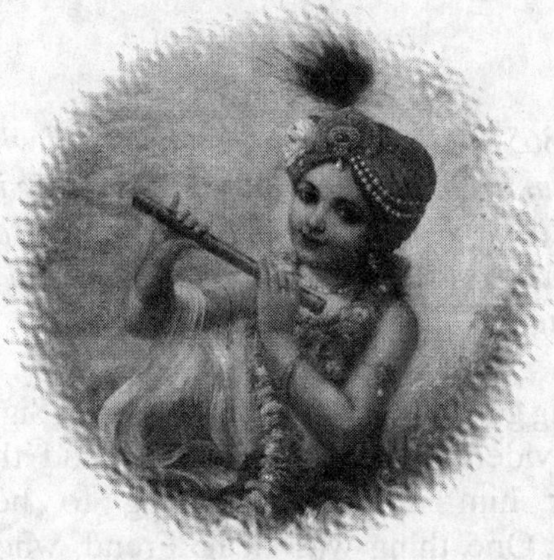

6.

Discussions on Western Philosophy And Science

Carl Jung: Seeker Without a Guide

Carl Jung (1865–1961) was a student of Freud who broke with him and began his own school of psychiatry. He is best known for his work in exploring the unconscious and for championing the importance of philosophy, religion, and mysticism in understanding the human mind.

Disciple: Jung gave the following criticism of Sigmund Freud: "Sexuality evidently meant more to Freud than to other people. For him it was something to be religiously observed. . . . One thing was clear: Freud, who had always made much of his irreligiosity, had now constructed a dogma. Or rather, in the place of a jealous God whom he had lost, he had substituted another compelling image, that of sexuality."
Śrīla Prabhupāda: Yes, that is a fact. He has taken sexuality to be God. It is our natural tendency to accept a leader, and Freud simply abandoned the leadership of God and took up the leadership of sex. On the other hand, if we accept the leadership of Kṛṣṇa, our life becomes perfect. All other leadership is the leadership of *māyā* [illusion]. There is no doubt that we have to accept a leader. Although Freud would not admit it, he accepted sex as his leader, and consequently he was constantly speaking about sex. Those who have taken God as their leader will speak only of God, nothing else. *Jīvera 'svarūpa' haya—kṛṣṇera 'nitya-dāsa'.* According to Caitanya Mahāprabhu's philosophy, we are all eternal servants of God, but as soon as we give up God's service, we have to accept the service of *māyā.*
Disciple: Jung sees the mind as being composed of a balance of the conscious and the unconscious, or subconscious. It is the function of the personality to integrate these. For instance, if one has a strong sex drive, he can sublimate or channel it into art or religious activity.
Śrīla Prabhupāda: That is our process. The sex impulse is natural for everyone in the material world. But if we think of

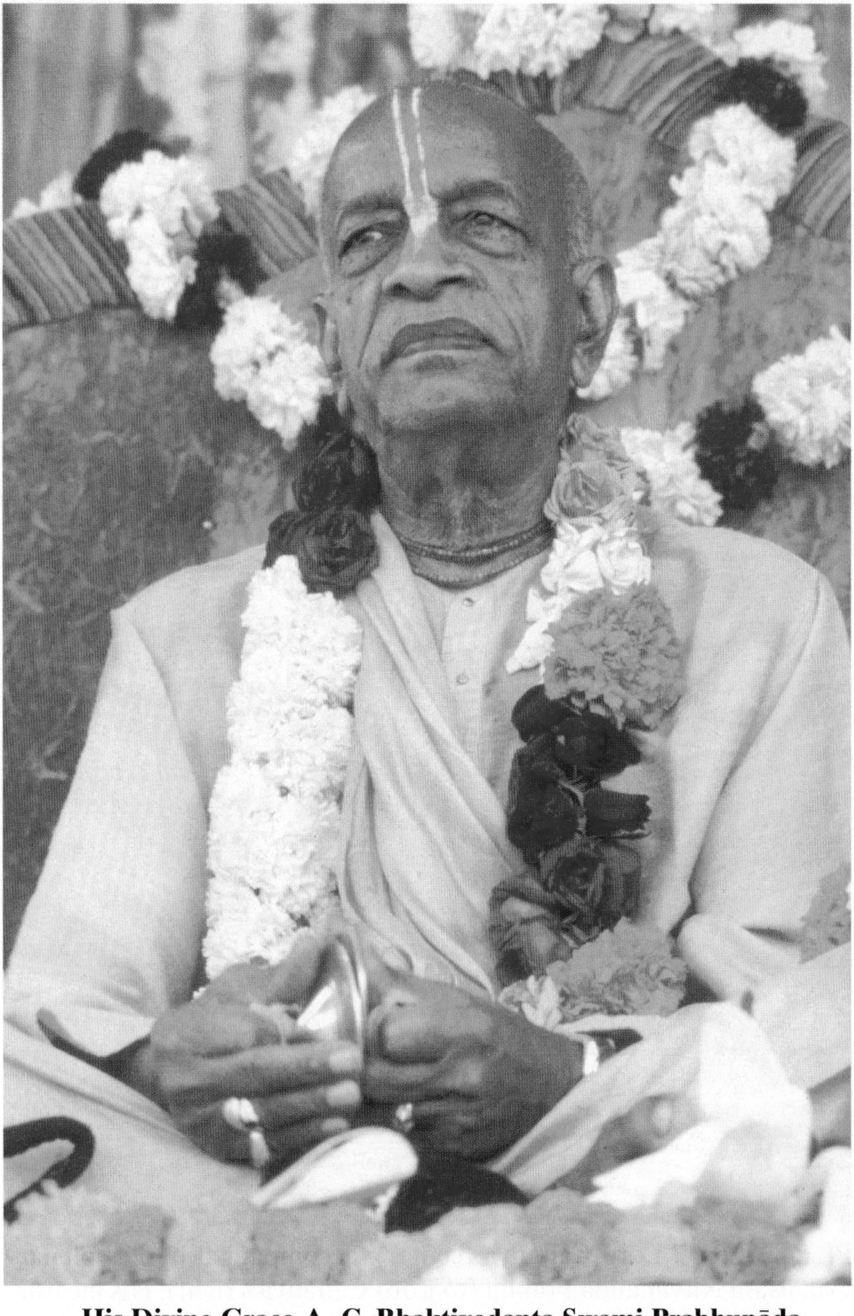

His Divine Grace A. C. Bhaktivedanta Swami Prabhupāda
*The Founder-*Ācārya *of the International Society for Krishna Consciousness and the greatest exponent of* Kṛṣṇa *consciousness in the modern world.*

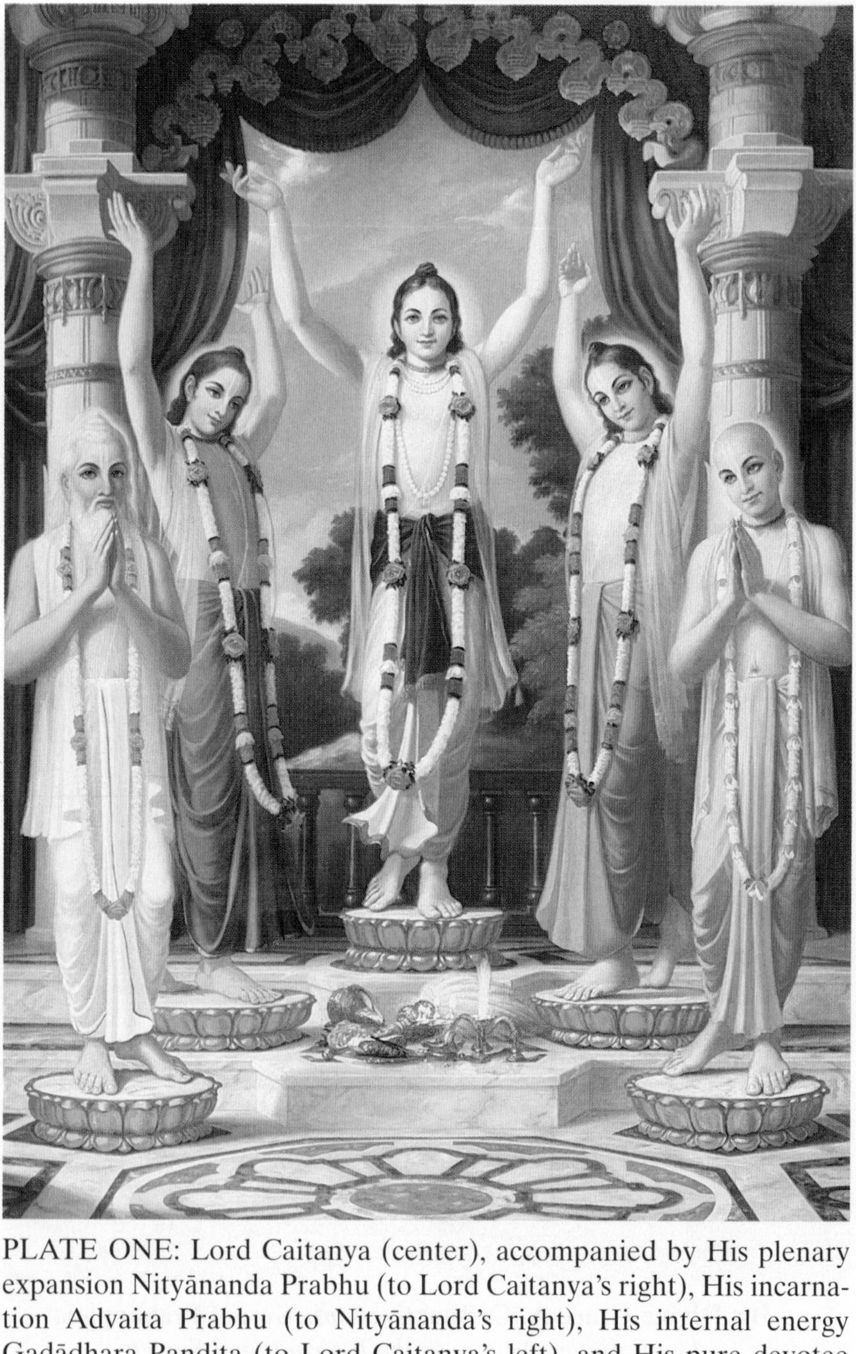

PLATE ONE: Lord Caitanya (center), accompanied by His plenary expansion Nityānanda Prabhu (to Lord Caitanya's right), His incarnation Advaita Prabhu (to Nityānanda's right), His internal energy Gadādhara Paṇḍita (to Lord Caitanya's left), and His pure devotee Śrīvāsa Ṭhākura. Together they spread love of Godhead through the chanting of the Hare Kṛṣṇa *mantra*. (*p.* 115)

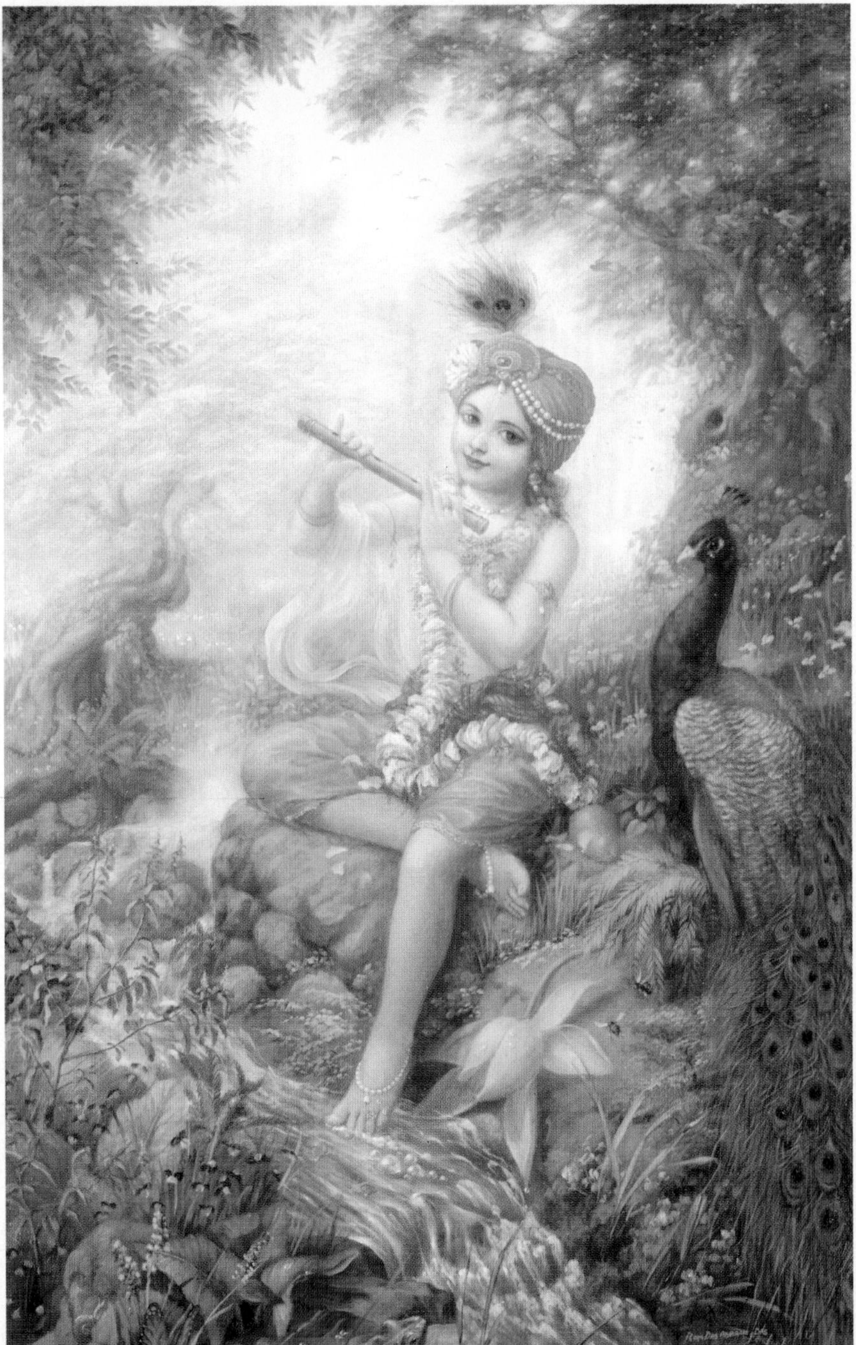

PLATE TWO: When Kṛṣṇa plays His flute in the forest of Vṛndāvana, all animate and inanimate beings become jubilant. (*p.* 48)

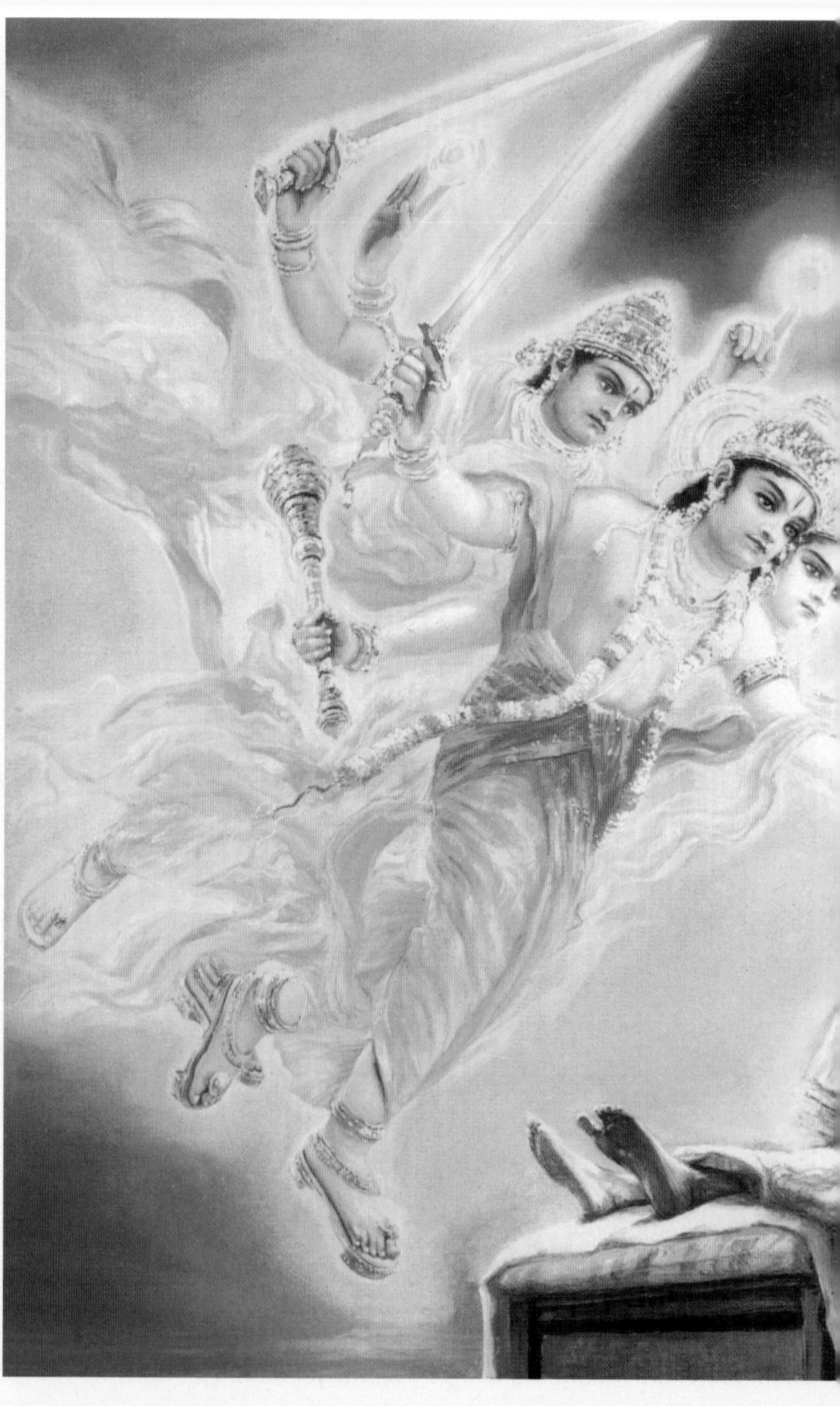

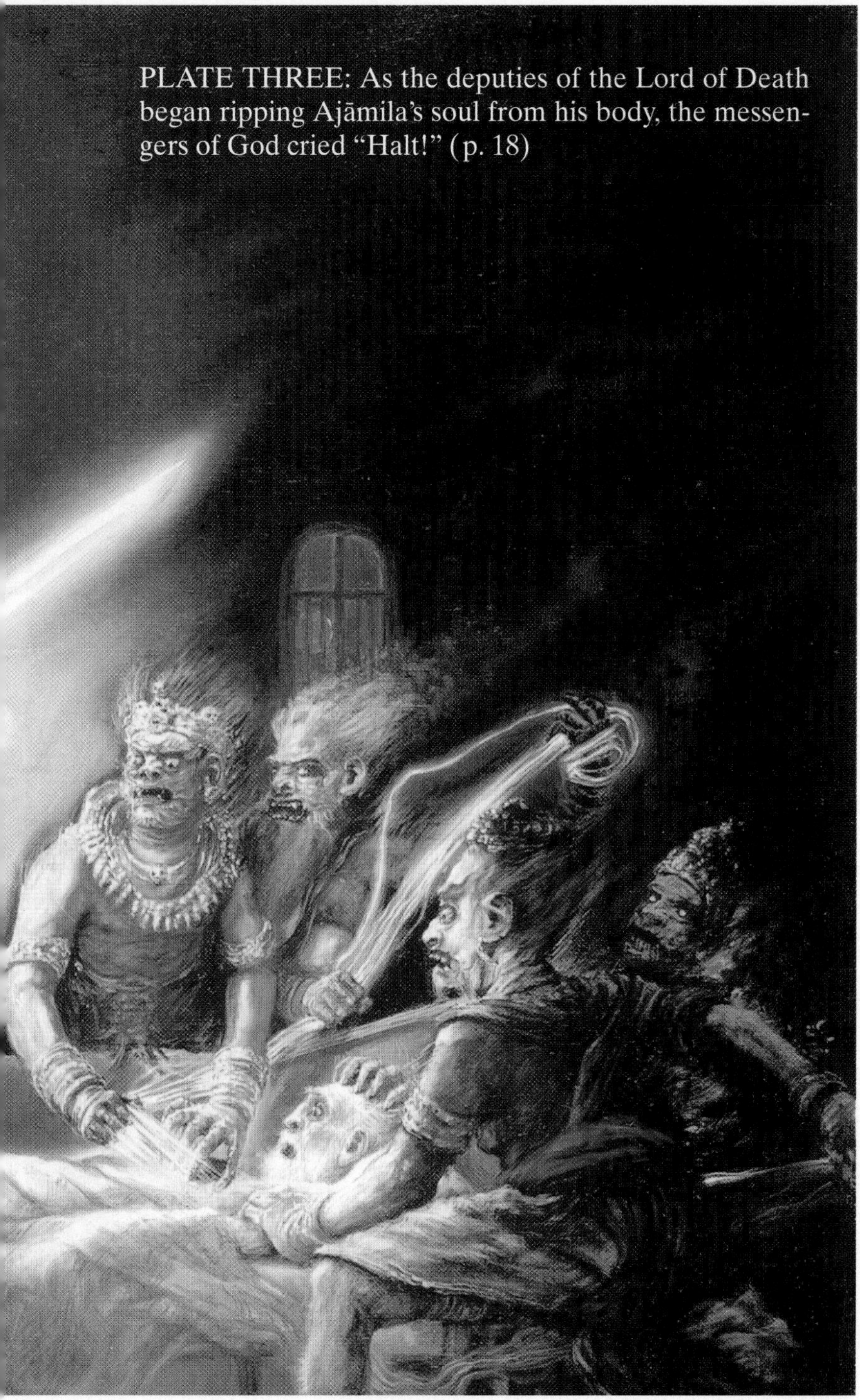

PLATE THREE: As the deputies of the Lord of Death began ripping Ajāmila's soul from his body, the messengers of God cried "Halt!" (p. 18)

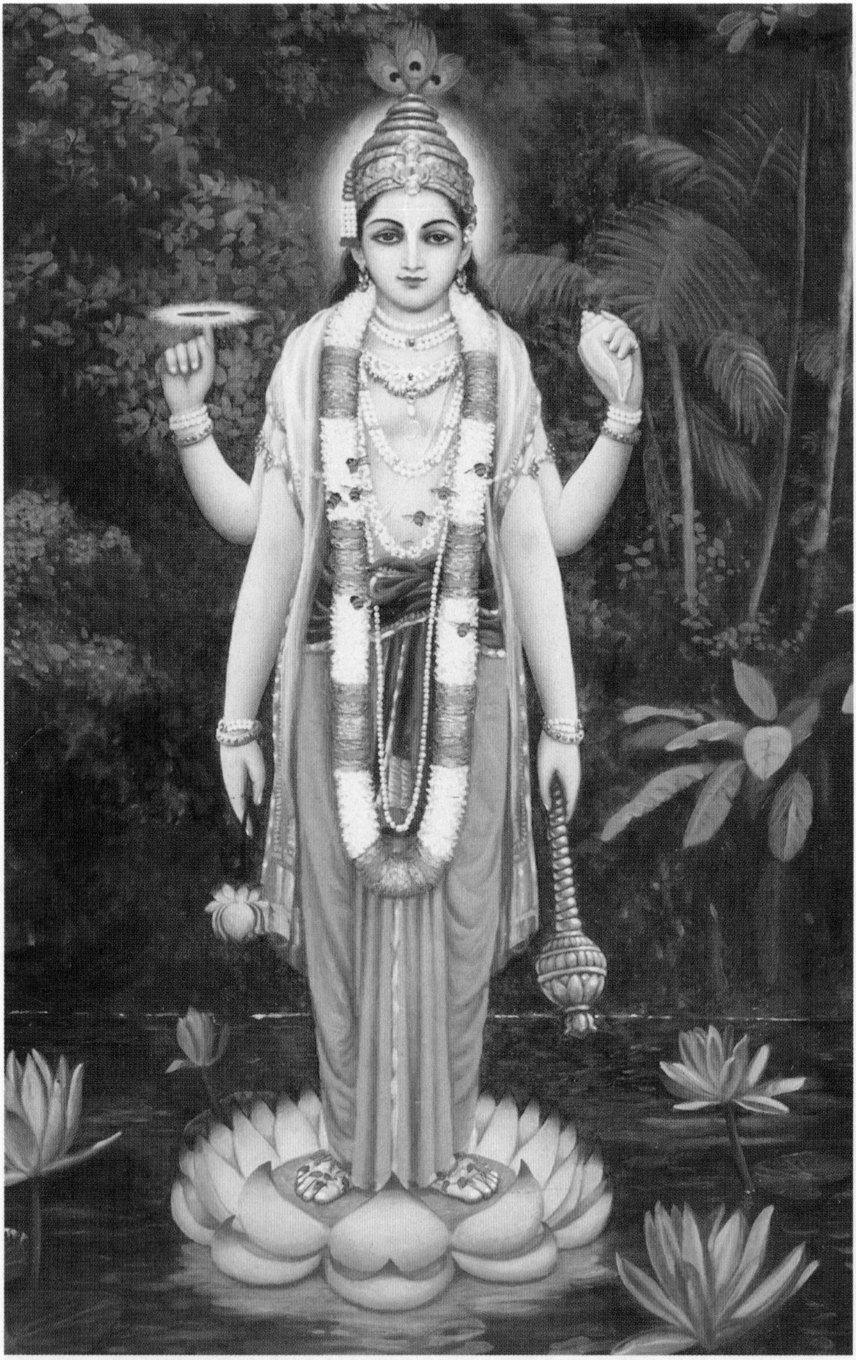

PLATE FOUR: Within the lake of everyone's heart resides a four-armed expansion of Kṛṣṇa known as the Supersoul. (*p.* 61)

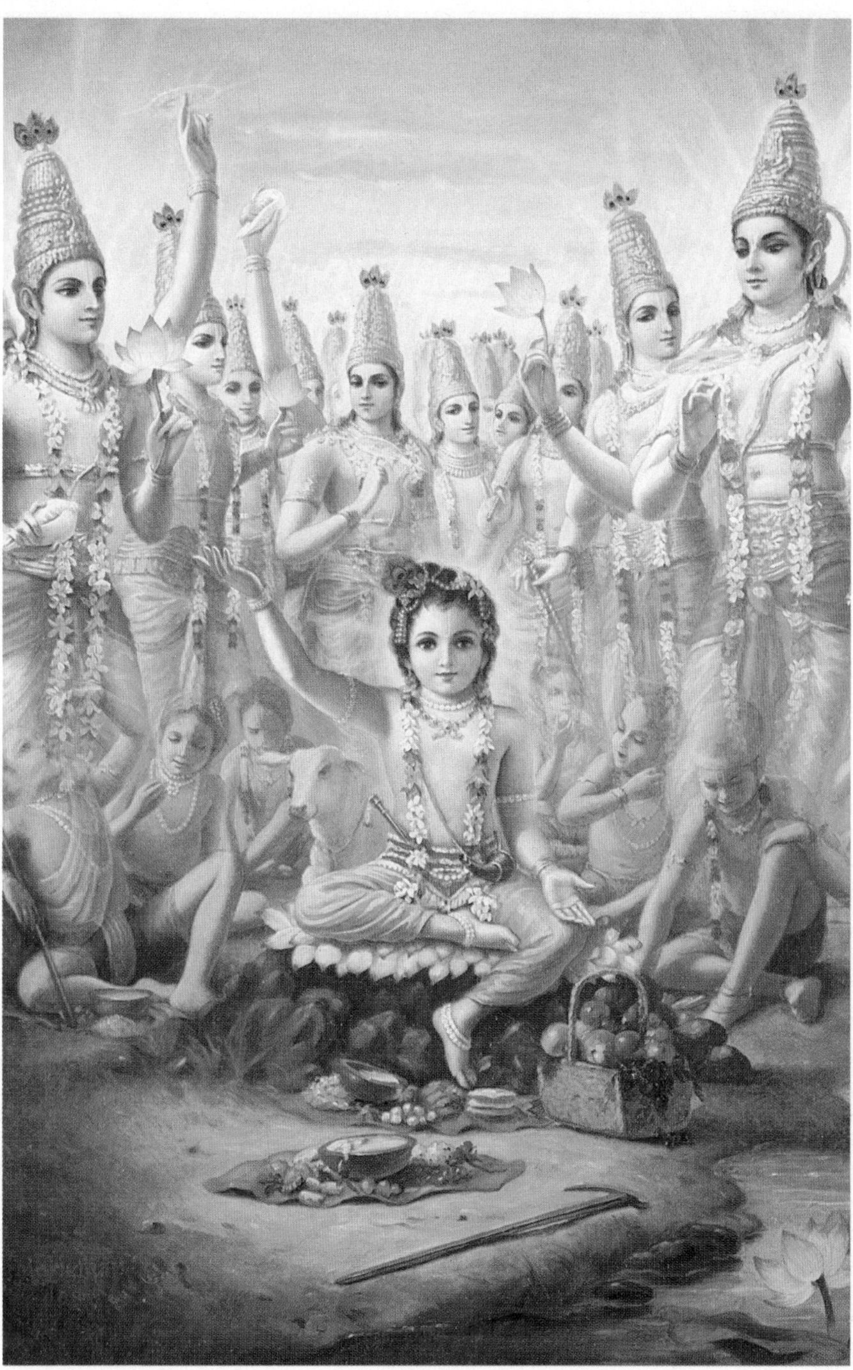

PLATE FIVE: Lord Kṛṣṇa can expand Himself into any number of plenary forms, called *viṣṇu-tattva*. (*p*. 172)

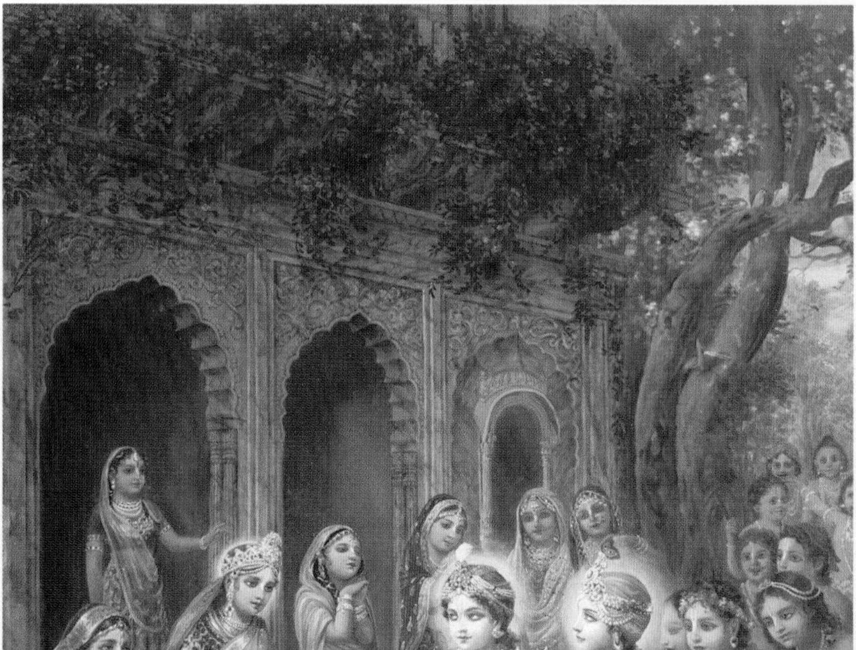

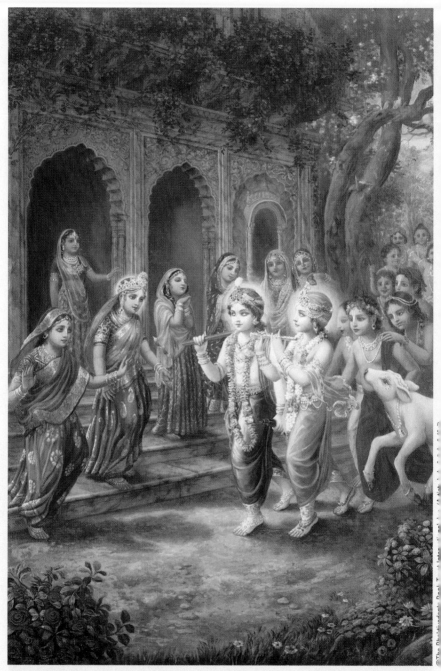

PLATE SIX: As Kṛṣṇa returns from the forest of Vṛndāvana in the evening, His cowherd girlfriends rush out to greet Him, overwhelmed with love. (*p.* 230)

Kṛṣṇa embracing Rādhārāṇī or dancing with the *gopīs,* our sex impulse is sublimated and weakened. If one hears about the pastimes of Kṛṣṇa and the *gopīs* from the right source, lusty desire within the heart will be suppressed, and one will be able to develop devotional service.

Disciple: This would be an example of what Jung would call integration or individuation, whereby the energies of the subconscious sex impulse are channeled into conscious, creative activity directed toward God realization.

Śrīla Prabhupāda: What we must understand is that Kṛṣṇa is the only *puruṣa,* the only enjoyer. If we help Him in His enjoyment, we also receive enjoyment. We are predominated, and He is the predominator. On the material platform, if a husband wants to enjoy the wife, the wife must voluntarily help him in that enjoyment. By helping him, the wife also becomes an enjoyer. Similarly, the supreme predominator, the supreme enjoyer, is Kṛṣṇa. And the predominated, the enjoyed, are the living entities. When the living entities agree to help Kṛṣṇa's sex desire, they become enjoyers.

Disciple: What is meant by Kṛṣṇa's sex desire?

Śrīla Prabhupāda: You might say "sense enjoyment." Kṛṣṇa is the supreme proprietor of the senses, and when we help Kṛṣṇa in His sense enjoyment, we also naturally partake of that enjoyment. The sweet *rasagullā* [a confection made from milk] is meant to be enjoyed, and therefore the hand puts it into the mouth so that it can be tasted and go to the stomach The hand cannot enjoy the *rasagullā* directly. Kṛṣṇa is the only direct enjoyer; all others are indirect enjoyers. By satisfying Kṛṣṇa, others will be satisfied. Upon seeing the predominator happy, the predominated become happy.

Disciple: Psychologists say that quite often the subconscious is acting through the conscious, but that we do not know it.

Śrīla Prabhupāda: Yes. The subconscious is there, but it is not always manifest. Sometimes a thought suddenly becomes manifest, just as a bubble will suddenly emerge in a pond. You may not know why it emerges, but we may assume that it was in the subconscious state and suddenly became manifest.

That subconscious thought which is manifest does not necessarily have any connection with one's present consciousness. It is like a stored impression, a shadow or a photograph. The mind takes many snapshots, and they are stored.

Disciple: Jung could see that the soul is always longing for light, and he wrote of the urge within the soul to rise out of darkness. He noted the pent-up feeling in the eyes of primitive people and a certain sadness in the eyes of animals. He wrote, "There is a sadness in animals' eyes, and we never know whether that sadness is bound up with the soul of the animal or is a poignant message which speaks to us out of that existence."

Śrīla Prabhupāda: Yes. Every living entity, including man, is constitutionally a servant. Therefore everyone is seeking some master, and that is our natural propensity. You can often see a puppy attempt to take shelter of some boy or man, and that is his natural tendency. He is saying, "Give me shelter. Keep me as your friend." A child or a man also wants some shelter in order to be happy. That is our constitutional position. When we attain the human form, when our consciousness is developed, we should take Kṛṣṇa as our shelter and our leader. In the *Bhagavad-gītā* Kṛṣṇa tells us that if we want shelter and guidance, we should take His. *Sarva-dharmān parityajya mām ekaṁ śaraṇaṁ vraja.* This is the ultimate instruction of the *Bhagavad-gītā.*

Disciple: Jung would say that our understanding of Kṛṣṇa as the supreme father and the cause of all causes is an archetypal understanding shared by all humans. All people have the tendency to understand someone to be their supreme father and primal cause, and they will represent Him in different ways. The archetype, however, is the same.

Śrīla Prabhupāda: Yes, it is exactly the same. Kṛṣṇa, or God, is the supreme father. A father has many sons, and all men are sons of God, born of their father. This is an experience common to everyone at all times.

Disciple: Jung believed that because there are so many subconscious factors governing our personality, we must awaken to them. Unless we do so, we are more or less slaves to our subconscious life. The point of psychoanalysis is to reveal as many aspects of our subconscious life as possible and enable us to face them.

Śrīla Prabhupāda: That is what we are teaching. We say that presently the soul is in a sleeping state, and we are telling the soul, "Please wake up! Please wake up! You are not this body! You are not this body!" It is possible to awaken the human being, but other living entities cannot be awakened. A tree, for instance, has consciousness, but he is so packed in matter that you cannot raise him to Kṛṣṇa consciousness. A human being, on the other hand, has developed consciousness, which is manifest in different stages. Lower life forms are more or less in a dream state.

Disciple: Whereas Freud was sexually oriented, Jung was more or less spiritually oriented. In his autobiography—*Memories, Dreams, Reflections*—Jung writes, "I find that all my thoughts circle around God like the planets around the sun, and are as irresistibly attracted by Him. I would feel it to be the grossest sin if I were to put up any resistance to this force." Jung sees all creatures as parts of God and at the same time unique in themselves. He writes, "Man cannot compare himself with any other creature; he is not a monkey, not a cow, not a tree. I am a man. But what is it to be that? Like every other being, I am a splinter of the infinite Deity. . . ."

Śrīla Prabhupāda: It is also our philosophy that we are part and parcel of God, just as sparks are part of a fire.

Disciple: Jung further writes in his autobiography, "It was obedience which brought me grace. . . . One must be utterly abandoned to God; nothing matters but fulfilling His will. Otherwise, all is folly and meaningless."

Śrīla Prabhupāda: Very good. Surrender unto God is real spiritual life. *Sarva-dharmān parityajya.* Surrender to God means accepting that which is favorable to God and rejecting that which is unfavorable. The devotee is always convinced that God will give him all protection. He remains humble and meek and thinks himself as one of the members of God's family. This is real spiritual communism. Communists think, "I am a member of a certain community," but it is a man's duty to think, "I am a member of God's family." God is the supreme father, material nature is the mother, and living entities are all sons of God. There are living entities everywhere—on land and in the air and water. There is no doubt that material nature is the mother, and according to our experience we can understand that a mother cannot produce a child without a father. It is absurd to think that a child can be born without a father. A father must be there, and the supreme father is God. In Kṛṣṇa consciousness, a person understands that the creation is a spiritual family headed by one supreme father.

Disciple: Concerning God's personality, Jung writes this: "According to the Bible, God has a personality and is the ego of the universe, just as I myself am the ego of my psychic and physical being."

Śrīla Prabhupāda: Yes. The individual is conscious of his own body, but not of the bodies of others. Besides the individual soul or consciousness in the body, there is the Paramātmā, the Supersoul, the superconsciousness present in everyone's heart. This is discussed in *Bhagavad-gītā* [13.3]:

kṣetra-jñaṁ cāpi māṁ viddhi sarva-kṣetreṣu bhārata
kṣetra-kṣetrajñayor jñānaṁ yat taj jñānaṁ mataṁ mama

"You should understand that I am also the knower in all bodies, and to understand this body and its knower is called knowledge."

Disciple: Recalling his difficulties in understanding God's personality, Jung writes, "Here I encountered a formidable obstacle. Personality, after all, surely signifies character. Now, character is one thing and not another; that is to say, it involves certain specific attributes. But if God is everything, how can He still possess a distinguishable character? . . . What kind of character or what kind of personality does He have?"

Śrīla Prabhupāda: God's character is transcendental, not material, and thus He has attributes. For instance, He is very kind to His devotee, and this kindness may be considered one of His characteristics or attributes. Whatever qualities or characteristics we have are but minute manifestations of God's. God is the origin of all attributes and characteristics. As indicated in the *śāstra* [scriptures], He also has mind, senses, feelings, sense perception, sense gratification, and everything else. Everything is there unlimitedly, and since we are part and parcel of God, we possess His qualities in minute quantities. The original qualities are in God and are manifest minutely in ourselves.

According to the *Vedas* God is a person, but His personality is unlimited. Just as my consciousness is limited to this body and His consciousness is the superconsciousness within every body, so I am a person confined to this particular body and He is the superperson living within all. As Kṛṣṇa tells Arjuna in the *Bhagavad-gītā* [2.12], the personality of God and the personalities of the individual souls are eternally existing. Kṛṣṇa tells Arjuna on the battlefield, "Never was there a time when I did not exist, nor you, nor all these kings, nor in the future shall any of us cease to be." Both God and the living entity are eternally persons, but God's personality is unlimited and the individual's personality is limited. God has unlimited power, wealth, fame, knowledge, beauty, and renunciation. We have limited, finite power, knowledge, fame, and so on. That is the difference between the two personalities.

Disciple:: Jung found that philosophies and theologies could not give him a clear picture of God's personality. He writes this: "'What is wrong with these philosophers?' I wondered—evidently, they know of God only by hearsay."

Śrīla Prabhupāda: Yes, that is also our complaint. The philosophers we have studied have failed to give any clear idea of God. Because they are speculating, they cannot give concrete, clear information. As far as we are concerned, our understanding of God is clear because we simply receive the information given to the world by God Himself. Kṛṣṇa is accepted as the Supreme Person by Vedic authorities; therefore we should have no reason not to accept Him as such. Nārāyaṇa, Lord Śiva, and Lord Brahmā possess different percentages of God's attributes, but Kṛṣṇa possesses all the attributes cent percent, in totality. Rūpa Gosvāmī has analyzed this in his *Bhakti-rasāmṛta-sindhu,* which we have translated as *The Nectar of Devotion.*

In any case, God is a person, and if we study man's attributes, we can also know something of God's. Just as we enjoy ourselves with friends, parents, and others, God also enjoys Himself in various relationships. There are five primary and seven secondary relationships that the living entities can have with God. Since the living entities take pleasure in these relationships, God is described as *akhila-rasāmṛta-sindhu,* the reservoir of all pleasure. There is no need to speculate about God or to try to imagine Him. The process for understanding is described by Lord Kṛṣṇa in the *Bhagavad-gītā* [7.1]:

mayy āsakta-manāḥ pārtha yogaṁ yuñjan mad-āśrayaḥ
asaṁśayaṁ samagraṁ māṁ yathā jñāsyasi tac chṛṇu

"Now hear, O Arjuna, how by practicing yoga in full consciousness of Me, with mind attached to Me, you can know Me in full, free from doubt." You can learn about God by always keeping yourself under His protection, or under the protection of His representative. Then without a doubt you can perfectly understand God; otherwise there is no question of understanding Him.

Disciple: Jung goes on to point out the difference between theologians and philosophers. He writes, "At least they [the theologians] are sure that God exists, even though they make contradictory statements about Him. . . . God's existence does not depend on our proofs. . . . I understand that God was, for me at least, one of the most certain and immediate of experiences."

Śrīla Prabhupāda: Yes, that is a transcendental conviction. One may not know God, but it is very easy to understand that God is there. One has to learn about God's nature, but there is no doubt about the fact that God is there. Any sane man can understand that he is being controlled. So who is that controller? The supreme controller is God. This is the conclusion of a sane man. Jung is right when he says that God's existence does not depend on our proof.
Disciple: Jung continues to recall his early spiritual quests in this way: "In my darkness . . . I could have wished for nothing better than a real, live guru, someone possessing superior knowledge and ability, who would have disentangled me from the involuntary creations of my imagination."
Śrīla Prabhupāda: Yes. According to the Vedic instructions, in order to acquire perfect knowledge, one must have a guru. *Tad vijñānārthaṁ sa gurum evābhigacchet.* The guru must factually be a representative of God. He must have seen and experienced God in fact, not simply in theory. We have to approach such a guru, and by service, surrender, and sincere inquiry we can come to understand God. The *Vedas* inform us that a person can understand God when he has received a little mercy from His Lordship; otherwise, one may speculate for millions and millions of years. As Kṛṣṇa states in the *Bhagavad-gītā* [18.55], *bhaktyā mām abhijānāti:* "One can understand Me as I am, as the Supreme Personality of Godhead, only by devotional service." This process of *bhakti* includes *śravaṇaṁ kīrtanaṁ viṣṇoḥ*—hearing and chanting about Lord Viṣṇu [Kṛṣṇa] and always remembering Him. *Satataṁ kīrtayanto māṁ:* the devotee is always glorifying the Lord. As Prahlāda Mahārāja says in *Śrīmad-Bhāgavatam* [7.9.43]:

naivodvije para duratyaya-vaitaraṇyās
tvad-vīrya-gāyana-mahāmṛta-magna-cittaḥ

"O best of the great personalities, I am not at all afraid of material existence, for wherever I stay I am fully absorbed in thoughts of Your glories and activities." The devotee's consciousness is always drowned in the ocean of the unlimited pastimes and qualities of the Supreme Lord. That is transcendental bliss. The spiritual master teaches his disciple how to always remain in the ocean of God consciousness. One who works under the directions of the *ācārya,* the spiritual master, knows everything about God.

Disciple: In 1938 Jung was invited by the British government to participate in celebrations at the University of Calcutta. Of this Jung writes, "By that time, I had read a great deal about Indian philosophy and religious history and was deeply convinced of the value of Oriental wisdom." On this visit, Jung spoke with a celebrated guru, yet he avoided so-called holy men. He writes, "I did so because I had to make do with my own truth, not to accept from others what I could not attain on my own. I would have felt it as a theft had I attempted to learn from the holy men to accept their truth for myself."

Śrīla Prabhupāda: On the one hand, he says he wants a guru, and then on the other, he doesn't want to accept one. Doubtlessly there were many so-called gurus in Calcutta, and Jung might have seen some bogus gurus he did not like. In any case, the principle of accepting a guru cannot be avoided. It is absolutely necessary.

Disciple: Concerning consciousness after death, Jung feels that after death the individual must pick up at the level of consciousness which he left.

Śrīla Prabhupāda: Yes, and therefore, according to that consciousness, one has to accept a body. That is the process of the soul's transmigration. An ordinary person can see only the gross material body, but accompanying this body are the mind, intelligence, and ego. When the body is finished, these remain, although they cannot be seen. A foolish man thinks that everything is finished at death. But the soul carries with it the mind, intelligence, and ego—that is, the subtle body—into another body. This is confirmed by the *Bhagavad-gītā,* which clearly explains that although the body is destroyed the consciousness continues. According to one's consciousness, one acquires another body, and again, in that body, the consciousness begins to mold its future lives. If a person was a devotee in his past life, he will again become a devotee after his death. Once the material body is destroyed, the same consciousness begins to work in another body. Consequently we find that some people quickly accept Kṛṣṇa consciousness whereas others take a longer time. This indicates that the consciousness is continuing, although the body is changing. Bharata Mahārāja, for instance, changed many bodies, but his consciousness continued, and he remained fully Kṛṣṇa conscious.

We may see a person daily, but we cannot visualize his intelligence. We can understand that a person is intelligent, but we cannot see intelligence itself. When one talks, we can understand that there is intelligence at work. But why should we conclude that when the gross body is dead and no longer capable of talking, the intelligence is finished? The instrument for speech is the gross body, but we should not conclude that when the gross body is finished, intelligence is also finished. *Na hanyate hanyamāne śarīre:* after the destruction of the gross body, the mind and intelligence continue. Because they require a body to function, they develop a body, and that is the process of the soul's transmigration.

Disciple: Jung felt that the individual's level of consciousness could not supersede whatever knowledge is available on this planet.

Śrīla Prabhupāda: No. One can supersede it, provided one can acquire knowledge from the proper authority. You may not have seen India, but a person who *has* seen India can describe it to you. We may not be able to see Kṛṣṇa, but we can learn of Him from an authority who knows. In the *Bhagavad-gītā* [8.20] Kṛṣṇa tells Arjuna that there is an eternal nature. On this earth we encounter temporary nature. Here things take birth, remain for some time, change, grow old, and are finally destroyed. There is dissolution in this material world, but there is another world, in which there is no dissolution. We have no personal experience of that world, but we can understand that it exists when we receive information from the proper authority. It is not necessary to know it by personal experience. There are different stages of knowledge, and not all knowledge can be acquired by direct perception. That is not possible.

Disciple: Jung sees earthly life to be of great significance, and what a man carries with him at the time of his death to be very important. He writes, "Only here, in life on earth, can the general level of consciousness be raised. That seems to be man's metaphysical task." Since consciousness survives death, it is important that a man's consciousness be elevated while he is on this earth.

Śrīla Prabhupāda: Yes, one's consciousness should be developed. As stated in the *Bhagavad-gītā,* if one's yoga practice is incomplete or if one dies prematurely, his consciousness accompanies him, and in the next life he begins at the point where he left off. His intelligence is revived. *Tatra taṁ buddhi-saṁyogaṁ labhate paurva-dehikam* [*Bhagavad-gītā* 6.43]. In an ordinary class we can see that some students learn very quickly while others cannot understand. This is evidence for the continuation of consciousness. If one is extraordinarily intelligent, the consciousness he developed in a previous life is being revived. The fact that we have undergone previous births is also evidence for the immortality of the soul.

Disciple: Jung points out that there is a paradox surrounding death. From the viewpoint of the ego, death is a horrible catastrophe—"a fearful piece of brutality." Yet from the viewpoint of the psyche—the soul—death is "a joyful event. In the light of eternity, it is a wedding."

Śrīla Prabhupāda: Yes, death is horrible for one who is going to accept a lower form of life, and it is a pleasure for the devotee, because he is returning home, back to Godhead.

Disciple: So death is not always joyful for the soul?

Śrīla Prabhupāda: No. How can it be? If one has not developed his spiritual consciousness—Kṛṣṇa consciousness—death is very horrible. The tendency in this life is to become very proud, and often people think, "I don't care for God. I am independent." Crazy people talk in this way, but after death they have to accept a body according to the dictations of nature. Nature says, "My dear sir, since you have worked like a dog, you can become a dog," or, "Since you have been surfing in the sea, you can now become a fish." These bodies are awarded according to a superior order. *Karmaṇā daiva-netreṇa.* In whatever way we interact with the modes of material nature, in that way we are creating our next body. How can we stop this process? This is nature's way.

If we are infected by some disease, we will necessarily get that disease. There are three modes of material nature—*tamo-guṇa, rajo-guṇa,* and *sattva-guṇa* [the modes of ignorance, passion, and goodness]—and our bodies are acquired according to our association with them. In general, the human form affords us a chance to make progress in Kṛṣṇa consciousness, especially when we are born in an aristocratic family, a *brāhmaṇa* [intellectual] family, or a Vaiṣṇava [devotee] family.

Disciple: Despite his many interesting points, Jung seems to have had a limited understanding of Indian philosophy. He does not understand that *saṁsāra* [the cycle of birth and death] has a goal, although it appears to be endless. Nor does he seem to know of Kṛṣṇa's promise in the *Bhagavad-gītā* that man can overcome earthly existence by surrendering unto Him.

Śrīla Prabhupāda: Overcoming earthly existence means entering into the spiritual world. The spirit soul is eternal, and it can enter from this atmosphere into another. Kṛṣṇa clearly explains this in the *Bhagavad-gītā* [4.9]:

janma karma ca me divyam evaṁ yo vetti tattvataḥ
tyaktvā dehaṁ punar janma naiti mām eti so 'rjuna

"One who knows the transcendental nature of My appearance and activities does not, upon leaving the body, take his birth again in this material world, but attains My eternal abode, O Arjuna." Those who continue to revolve in the cycle of birth and death acquire one material body after another, but those who are Kṛṣṇa conscious go to Kṛṣṇa. They do not acquire another material body.

Disciple: Śrī Kṛṣṇa says this repeatedly throughout *Bhagavad-gītā.*

Śrīla Prabhupāda: Yes, and those who are not envious of Kṛṣṇa accept His instructions, surrender unto Him, and understand Him. For them, this is the last material birth. For those who are envious, however, transmigration is continuous.

Disciple: Concerning *karma,* Jung writes this: "The crucial question is whether a man's *karma* is personal or not. If it is, then the preordained destiny with which a man enters life presents an achievement of previous lives, and a personal continuity therefore exists. If, however, this is not so, and an impersonal *karma* is seized upon in the act of birth, then that *karma* is incarnated again without there being any personal continuity."

Śrīla Prabhupāda: *Karma is* always personal.

Disciple: Jung goes on to point out that Buddha was twice asked by his disciples whether man's *karma* is personal or not, and each time he fended off the question and did not discuss the matter. To know this, the Buddha said, "would not contribute to liberating oneself from the illusion of existence."

Śrīla Prabhupāda: Buddha refused to answer because he did not teach about the soul or accept the personal soul. As soon as you deny the personal aspect of the soul, there is no question of a personal *karma.* Buddha wanted to avoid this question. He did not want his whole philosophy dismantled.

Disciple: Jung gives his own conclusion in this way: "Have I lived before in the past as a specific personality, and did I progress so far in that life that I am now able to seek a solution?"

Śrīla Prabhupāda: As we have mentioned earlier, that is explained in the *Bhagavad-gītā* [6.43]: *tatra taṁ buddhi-saṁyogaṁ labhate paurva-dehikam:* "On taking rebirth, one revives the consciousness of his previous life and tries to make further progress."

Disciple: Jung continues, "I imagine that I have lived in former centuries and there encountered questions I was not yet able to answer, that I had to be born again to fulfill the task that was given to me."

Śrīla Prabhupāda: That is a fact.

Disciple: "When I die, my deeds will follow along with me—that is how I imagine it."

Śrīla Prabhupāda: That is personal *karma*.

Disciple: Jung continues, "I will bring with me what I have done. In the meantime it is important to insure that I do not stand at the end with empty hands."

Śrīla Prabhupāda: If you are making regular progress in Kṛṣṇa consciousness, your hands will not be empty at the end. Completeness means returning home, back to Godhead. This return is not empty. A Vaiṣṇava does not want emptiness—eternal life with Kṛṣṇa is our aspiration. Materialists are thinking that at the end of life everything will be empty; therefore they conclude that they should enjoy themselves as much as possible in this life. That is why sense enjoyment is at the core of material life; materialists are mad after sense enjoyment.

Disciple: Jung believed that one is reborn due to *karma,* or selfish action. He wrote, "If *karma* still remains to be disposed of, then the soul relapses again into desires and returns to live once more, perhaps even doing so out of the realization that something remains to be completed. In my case, it must have been primarily a passionate urge toward understanding which brought about my birth, for that was the strongest element in my nature."

Śrīla Prabhupāda: That understanding for which he is longing is understanding of Kṛṣṇa. This Kṛṣṇa explains in the *Bhagavad-gītā* [7.19]:

bahūnāṁ janmanām ante jñānavān māṁ prapadyate
vāsudevaḥ sarvam iti sa mahātmā su-durlabhaḥ

One's understanding is complete when one comes to the point of understanding that Kṛṣṇa is everything. Then one's material journey comes to an end: *tyaktvā dehaṁ punar janma naiti* [*Bhagavad-gītā* 4.9]. When one's understanding of Kṛṣṇa is incomplete, Kṛṣṇa gives instructions by which one can understand Him completely. In the Seventh Chapter of the *Bhagavad-gītā* Kṛṣṇa says, *asaṁśayaṁ samagraṁ māṁ yathā jñāsyasi tac chṛnu:* "Now hear from Me how you can understand Me completely and without any doubt" [*Bhagavad-gītā* 7.1]. If we can understand Kṛṣṇa completely, we will take our next birth in the spiritual world.

Disciple: Jung conceived of a *persona,* which seems identical with what we call the false ego. He wrote, "The *persona* . . . is the individual's system of adaptation to, or the manner he assumes in dealing with, the world. A professor, for example, has his own characteristic *persona.* But the danger is that people become identical with their *personas*—the professor with his textbook, the tenor with his voice. One can say, with a little exaggeration, that the *persona* is that which in reality one is not, but which oneself as well as others think one is."

Śrīla Prabhupāda: One's real *persona* is that one is the eternal servant of God. This is the spiritual conception of life, and when one realizes this, his *persona* becomes his salvation and perfection. But as long as one is in the material conception of life, one's *persona* is that one is the servant of one's family, community, body, nation, ideal, and so on. In either case the *persona* is there and must continue, but proper understanding is realizing that one is the eternal servant of Kṛṣṇa. As long as one is in the material conception, one labors under the delusion of the false ego, thinking, "I am an American," "I am a Hindu," and so on. This is the false ego at work. In reality we are all servants of God. When we speak of a "false ego," we imply a real ego, a purified ego. One whose ego is purified understands that he is the servant of Kṛṣṇa.

Disciple: For Jung, the purpose of psychoanalysis is to come to grips with our subconscious, shadow personality. Then we can know completely who we are.

Śrīla Prabhupāda: That means attaining real knowledge. When Sanātana Gosvāmī approached Śrī Caitanya Mahāprabhu, Sanātana said, "Please reveal to me who and what I am." In order to understand our real identity, we require the assistance of a guru.
Disciple: Jung says that in the shadow personality of all males there is a bit of the female, and in all females there is a bit of the male. Because we repress these aspects of the shadow personality, we do not understand our actions.
Śrīla Prabhupāda: We say that every living entity is by nature a female, *prakṛti. Prakṛti* means "female," and *puruṣa* means "male." Although we are *prakṛti,* in this material world we are posing ourselves as *puruṣa.* Because the *jīvātmā,* the individual soul, has the propensity to enjoy as a male, he is sometimes described as *puruṣa.* But actually the *jīvātmā* is not *puruṣa.* He is *prakṛti. Prakṛti* means the predominated, and *puruṣa* means the predominator. The only predominator is Kṛṣṇa; therefore originally we are all female by constitution. But under illusion we attempt to become males, enjoyers. This is called *māyā.* Although a female by constitution, the living entity is trying to imitate the supreme male, Kṛṣṇa. When one comes to his original consciousness, one understands that he is not the predominator but the predominated.
Disciple: Jung wrote of the soul in this way: "If the human soul is anything, it must be of unimaginable complexity and diversity, so that it cannot possibly be approached through a mere psychology of instinct."
Śrīla Prabhupāda: According to Caitanya Mahāprabhu, we can understand the soul through training. We should understand that we are not *brāhmaṇas* [intellectuals], *kṣatriyas* [administrators], *sannyāsīs* [renunciants], *brahmacārīs* [celibate students], or whatever. By negation we can understand, "I am not this, I am not that." Then what *is* our identity? Caitanya Mahāprabhu says, *gopī-bhartuḥ pada-kamalayor dāsa-dāsānudāsaḥ:* "I am the servant of the servant of the servant of Kṛṣṇa, the maintainer of the *gopīs* [Kṛṣṇa's dearmost servants, the milkmaids of Vṛndāvana]." That is our real iden-

tity. As long as we do not identify ourselves as eternal servants of Kṛṣṇa, we will be subject to various false identifications. *Bhakti,* devotional service, is the means by which we can be purified of false identifications.

Disciple: Concerning the soul, Jung further wrote, "I can only gaze with wonder and awe at the depths and heights of our psychic nature. Its nonspatial universe conceals an untold abundance of images which have accumulated over millions of years. . . ."

Śrīla Prabhupāda: Since we are constantly changing our bodies, constantly undergoing transmigration, we are accumulating various experiences. However, if we remain fixed in Kṛṣṇa consciousness, we do not change. There is none of this fluctuation once we understand our real identity, which is, "I am the servant of Kṛṣṇa; my duty is to serve Him." Arjuna realized this after hearing the *Bhagavad-gītā,* and he told Śrī Kṛṣṇa,

naṣṭo mohaḥ smṛtir labdhā tvat-prasādān mayācyuta
sthito 'smi gata-sandehaḥ kariṣye vacanaṁ tava

"My dear Kṛṣṇa, O infallible one, my illusion is now gone. I have regained my memory by Your mercy, and I am now firm and free from doubt and am prepared to act according to Your instructions" [*Bhagavad-gītā* 18.73].

So after hearing the *Bhagavad-gītā* Arjuna comes to this conclusion, and his illusion is dispelled by Kṛṣṇa's mercy. Arjuna is then fixed in his original position. And what is this? *Kariṣye vacanaṁ tava:* "Whatever You say, I shall do." At the beginning of the *Bhagavad-gītā* Kṛṣṇa told Arjuna to fight, and Arjuna refused. At the conclusion of the *Bhagavad-gītā* Arjuna's illusion is dispelled, and he is situated in his original constitutional position. Thus our perfection lies in executing the orders of Kṛṣṇa.

Disciple: Jung noted that the world's religions speak of five different types of rebirth. One is metempsychosis, the transmigration of souls, and, according to this view, "one's life is prolonged in time by passing through different bodily existences; or, from another point of view, it is a life-sequence interrupted by different reincarnations. . . . It is by no means certain whether continuity of personality is guaranteed or not: there may be only a continuity of *karma*."

Śrīla Prabhupāda: A personality is always there, and bodily changes do not affect it. However, one identifies himself according to his body. For instance, when the soul is within the body of a dog, he thinks according to that particular bodily construction. He thinks, "I am a dog, and I have my particular activities." In human society the same conception is there. For instance, when one is born in America he thinks, "I am an American, and I have my duty." According to the body, the personality is manifest—but in all cases personality is there.

Disciple: But is this personality continuous?

Śrīla Prabhupāda: Certainly the personality is continuous. At death the soul passes into another gross body along with its mental and intellectual identifications. The individual acquires different types of bodies, but the person is the same.

Disciple: This would correspond to the second type of rebirth, which is reincarnation. Jung wrote, "This concept of rebirth necessarily implies the continuity of personality. Here the human personality is regarded as continuous and accessible to memory, so that when one is incarnated or born, one is able, at least potentially, to remember that one has lived through previous existences and that these existences were one's own—that is, that they had the same ego-form as the present life. As a rule, reincarnation means rebirth into a human body."

Śrīla Prabhupāda: Not necessarily into a human body. From *Śrīmad-Bhāgavatam* we learn that Bharata Mahārāja became a deer in his next life. The soul is changing bodies just as a man changes his clothes. The man is the same, although his clothes may be different:

vāsāṁsi jīrṇāni yathā vihāya
navāni gṛhṇāti naro 'parāṇi

tathā śarīrāṇi vihāya jīrṇāny
anyāni saṁyāti navāni dehī

"As a person puts on new garments, giving up old ones, the soul similarly accepts new material bodies, giving up the old and useless ones" [*Bhagavad-gītā* 2.22]. When a coat is old and cannot be used anymore, one has to purchase another. The man is the same, but his clothes are supplied according to the price he can pay. Similarly, you "purchase" a new body with the "money" (*karma*) you have accumulated in your life. According to your *karma,* you receive a certain type of body.

Disciple: The third type of rebirth is called resurrection, and Jung notes that there are two types of resurrection. "It may be a carnal body, as in the Christian assumption that this body will be resurrected." According to the Christian doctrine, at the end of the world the gross bodies will reassemble themselves and ascend into heaven or descend into hell.

Śrīla Prabhupāda: This is simply foolishness. The gross material body can never be resurrected. At the time of death the living entity leaves this material body, and the material body disintegrates. How can the material elements reassemble themselves?

Disciple: Jung further wrote that on a higher level resurrection is no longer understood in a gross material sense: "It is assumed that the resurrection of the dead is the raising up of the *corpus gloriaficationis,* the subtle body, in the state of incorruptibility."

Śrīla Prabhupāda: This type of "resurrection" is applicable only to God and His representatives, not to others. In this case, it is not a material body that is "raised up," but a spiritual one. When God appears, he appears in a spiritual body, and this body does not change. In the *Bhagavad-gītā* Kṛṣṇa says that he spoke to the sun-god millions of years ago, and Arjuna questions how this could be possible. Kṛṣṇa replies that although Arjuna had been present he could not remember. It is possible for one to remember only if one does not change bodies—changing bodies means forgetting. But the

Lord's body is purely spiritual, and a spiritual body never changes. According to the Māyāvādī conception, the Absolute Truth is impersonal, and when He appears as a person He accepts a material body. But those who are advanced in spiritual knowledge, who accept the *Bhagavad-gītā,* understand that this is not the case. Kṛṣṇa specifically says, *avajānanti māṁ mūḍhā mānuṣīṁ tanum āśritam:* "Because I appear as a human being, the unintelligent think that I am nothing but a human being" [*Bhagavad-gītā* 9.11]. This is not the case. Impersonalists have no knowledge of the spiritual body.

Disciple: The fourth form of rebirth is called renovation, and this applies to "the transformation of a mortal into an immortal being, of a corporeal into a spiritual being, and of a human into a divine being. Well-known prototypes of this change ore the transfiguration and ascension of Christ, and the bodily assumption of the mother of God into heaven after her death."

Śrīla Prabhupāda: We say that the spiritual body never dies but that the material body is subject to destruction. *Na hanyate hanyamāne śarīre:* the material body is subject to destruction, but after its destruction the spiritual body is still there. The spiritual body is neither generated nor killed.

Disciple: But aren't there examples in the *Śrīmad-Bhāgavatam* of a kind of ascension into heaven? Didn't Arjuna ascend?

Śrīla Prabhupāda: Yes, and Yudhiṣṭhira. There are many instances—especially Kṛṣṇa Himself and His associates. But we should never consider their bodies material. They didn't go through death of any sort, although their bodies traveled to the higher universe. But it is also a fact that everyone possesses a spiritual body.

Disciple: The fifth type of rebirth is indirect and is called "participation in the process of transformation." Examples of this type may be the initiation ceremony or the twice-born ceremony of the *brāhmaṇa.* "In other words," Jung wrote, "one has to witness, or take part in, some rite of transformation. This rite may be a ceremony. . . . Through his presence at the rite, the individual participates in divine grace."

Śrīla Prabhupāda: Yes, one's first birth is by one's father and mother, and the next birth is by the spiritual master and Vedic knowledge. When one takes his second birth, he comes to understand that he is not the material body. This is spiritual education. That birth of knowledge, or birth *into* knowledge, is called *dvija,* "second birth."

Disciple: Thus far we have discussed only Jung's autobiography. In one of Jung's last books, *The Undiscovered Self,* he discussed the meaning of religion and its utility in the modern world. He wrote, "The meaning and purpose of religion lie in the relationship of the individual to God (Christianity, Judaism, Islam) or to the path of salvation and liberation (Buddhism). From this basic fact all ethics is derived, which without the individual's responsibility before God can be called nothing more than conventional morality."

Śrīla Prabhupāda: First of all, we understand from the *Bhagavad-gītā* that no one can approach God without being purified of all sinful reactions. Only one who is standing on the platform of pure goodness can understand God and engage in His service. From Arjuna we understand that God is *paraṁ brahma paraṁ dhāma pavitraṁ paramaṁ bhavān:* He is "the Supreme Brahman, the ultimate, the supreme abode and purifier" [*Bhagavad-gītā* 10.12]. *Paraṁ brahma* indicates the Supreme Brahman. Every living being is Brahman, or spirit, but Kṛṣṇa is the *paraṁ brahma,* the Supreme Brahman. He is also *paraṁ dhāma,* the ultimate abode of everything. He is also *pavitraṁ paramam,* the purest of the pure. In order to approach the purest of the pure, one must become completely pure, and to this end morality and ethics are necessary. Therefore, in our Kṛṣṇa consciousness movement we prohibit illicit sex, meat-eating, intoxication, and gambling—the four pillars of sinful life. If we can avoid these sinful activities, we can remain on the platform of purity. Kṛṣṇa consciousness is based on this morality, and one who cannot follow these principles falls down from the spiritual platform.

Thus, purity is the basic principle of God consciousness and is essential for the re-establishment of our eternal relationship with God.

Disciple: Jung saw atheistic communism as the greatest threat in the world today. He wrote, "The communistic revolution has debased man far lower than democratic collective psychology has done, because it robs him of his freedom not only in the social but in the moral and spiritual sense. . . . The state has taken the place of God; that is why, seen from this angle, the socialist dictatorships are religious, and state slavery is a form of worship."

Śrīla Prabhupāda: Yes, I agree with him. Atheistic communism has contributed to the degradation of human civilization. The communists supposedly believe in the equal distribution of wealth. According to our understanding, God is the father, material nature is the mother, and the living entities are the sons. The sons have a right to live at the cost of the father. The entire universe is the property of the Supreme Personality of Godhead, and the living entities are being supported by the supreme father. However, one should be satisfied with the supplies allotted to him. According to the *Īśopaniṣad, tena tyaktena bhuñjīthāḥ:* we should be satisfied with our allotment and not envy one another or encroach upon one another's property. We should not envy the capitalists or the wealthy, because everyone is given his allotment by the Supreme Personality of Godhead. Consequently, everyone should be satisfied with what he receives.

On the other hand, one should not exploit others. One may be born in a wealthy family, but one should not interfere with the rights of others. Whether one is rich or poor, one should be God conscious, accept God's arrangement, and serve God to his fullest. This is the philosophy of *Śrīmad-Bhāgavatam,* and it is confirmed by Śrī Caitanya Mahāprabhu. We should be content with our allocations from God and concern ourselves with advancing in Kṛṣṇa consciousness. If we become envious of the rich, we will be tempted to encroach upon their allotment, and in this way we are diverted from our service to the Lord. The main point is that everyone, rich or poor, should engage in God's service. If everyone does so, there will be real peace in the world.

Disciple: Concerning the socialist state, Jung further wrote, "The goals of religion—deliverance from evil, reconciliation with God, rewards in the hereafter, and so on—turn into worldly promises about freedom from care for one's daily bread, the just distribution of material goods, universal prosperity in the future, and shorter working hours." In other words, the communists place emphasis on immediate tactile rewards.

Śrīla Prabhupāda: This is because they have no understanding of spiritual life, nor can they understand that the person within the body is eternal and spiritual. Therefore they recommend immediate sense gratification.

Disciple: Jung believed, however, that socialism or Marxism cannot possibly replace religion in the proper, traditional sense. "A natural function which has existed from the beginning—like the religious function—cannot be disposed of with rationalistic and so-called enlightened criticism."

Śrīla Prabhupāda: The communists are concerned with adjusting material things, which can actually never be adjusted. They imagine that they can solve problems, but ultimately their plans will fail. The communists do not understand what religion actually is. It is not possible to avoid religion. Everything has a particular characteristic. Salt is salty, sugar is sweet, and chili is hot or pungent. These are intrinsic characteristics. Similarly, the living entity has an intrinsic quality. His characteristic is to render service—be he a communist, a theist, a capitalist, or whatever. In all countries people are working and rendering service to their respective governments—be they capitalists or communists—and the people are not getting any lasting benefit. Therefore we say that if people follow in the footsteps of Śrī Caitanya Mahāprabhu by serving Kṛṣṇa, they will actually be happy. Both communists and capitalists are saying, "Render service to me," but Kṛṣṇa says, *sarva-dharmān parityajya:* "Just give up all other service and render service unto Me, and I will free you from all sinful reactions" [*Bhagavad-gītā* 18.66].

Disciple: Jung feels that materialistic Western capitalism cannot possibly defeat a pseudo religion like Marxism. He believes that the only way the individual can combat atheistic communism is to adopt a nonmaterialistic religion. He wrote, "It has been correctly realized in many quarters that the alexipharmic, the antidote, should in this case be an equally potent faith of a different and nonmaterialistic kind. . . ." So Jung sees modern man in desperate need of a religion that has immediate meaning. He feels that Christianity is no longer effective because it no longer expresses what modern man needs most.

Śrīla Prabhupāda: That nonmaterialistic religion which is above everything—Marxism or capitalism—is this Kṛṣṇa consciousness movement. Kṛṣṇa has nothing to do with any materialistic "ism," and this movement is directly connected with Kṛṣṇa, the Supreme Personality of Godhead. God demands complete surrender, and we are teaching, "You are servants, but your service is being wrongly placed. Therefore you are not happy. Just render service to Kṛṣṇa, and you will find happiness." We support neither communism nor capitalism, nor do we advocate the adoption of pseudo religions. We are only for Kṛṣṇa.

Disciple: Concerning the social situation, Jung wrote, "It is unfortunately only too clear that if the individual is not truly regenerated in spirit, society cannot be either, for society is the sum total of individuals in need of redemption."

Śrīla Prabhupāda: The basis of change is the individual. Now there are a few individuals initiated into Kṛṣṇa consciousness, and if a large percentage can thus become invigorated, the face of the world will change. There is no doubt of this.

Disciple: For Jung, the salvation of the world consists in the salvation of the individual soul. The only thing that saves man from submersion into the masses is his relationship to God. Jung wrote, "His individual relation to God would be an effective shield against these pernicious influences."

Śrīla Prabhupāda: Yes, those who take Kṛṣṇa consciousness seriously are never troubled by Marxism, this-ism, or that-ism. A Marxist may take to Kṛṣṇa consciousness, but a Kṛṣṇa conscious devotee would never become a Marxist. That is not possible. It is explained in the *Bhagavad-gītā* that one who knows the highest perfection of life cannot be misled by a third- or fourth-class philosophy.
Disciple: Jung also felt that materialistic progress could be a possible enemy to the individual. He wrote, "A [materially] favorable environment merely strengthens the dangerous tendency to expect everything to originate from outside—even that metamorphosis which external reality cannot provide, namely, a deep-seated change of the inner man. . . ."
Śrīla Prabhupāda: Yes, everything originates from inside, from the soul. It is confirmed by Bhaktivinoda Ṭhākura and others that material progress is essentially an expansion of the external energy—*māyā,* illusion. We are all living in illusion, and so-called scientists and philosophers can never understand God and their relationship to Him, despite their material advancement. Material advancement and knowledge are actually a hindrance to the progressive march of Kṛṣṇa consciousness. We therefore minimize our necessities to live a saintly life. We are not after luxurious living. We feel that life is meant for spiritual progress and Kṛṣṇa consciousness, not for material advancement.
Disciple: To inspire this deep-seated change in the inner man, Jung feels that a proper teacher is needed, someone to explain religion to man.
Śrīla Prabhupāda: Yes. According to the Vedic injunction, it is essential to seek out a guru—a person who is a representative of God. *Sākṣād-dharitvena samasta-śāstraiḥ.* The representative of God is worshiped as God, but he never says, "I am God." Although he is worshiped as God, he is the servant of God—God Himself is always the master. Caitanya Mahāprabhu requested everyone to become a guru: "Wherever you are, simply become a guru and deliver all these people who are in ignorance." One may say, "I am not very

learned. How can I become a guru?" But Caitanya Mahāprabhu said that it is not necessary to be a learned scholar, for there are many so-called learned scholars who are fools. It is only necessary to impart Kṛṣṇa's instructions, which are already there in the *Bhagavad-gītā.* Whoever explains the *Bhagavad-gītā* as it is—he is a guru. If one is fortunate enough to approach such a guru, his life becomes successful.

Disciple: Jung also laments the fact that "our philosophy is no longer a way of life, as it was in antiquity; it has turned into an exclusively intellectual and academic affair."

Śrīla Prabhupāda: That is also our opinion: mental speculation has no value in itself. One must be directly in touch with the Supreme Personality of Godhead, and using all reason, one must assimilate the instructions given by Him. One can then follow these instructions in one's daily life and do good to others by teaching *Bhagavad-gītā.*

Disciple: On one hand, Jung sees an exclusively intellectual philosophy; on the other, denominational religions with "archaic rites and conceptions" that "express a view of the world which caused no great difficulties in the Middle Ages, but which has become strange and unintelligible to the man of today."

Śrīla Prabhupāda: That is because preachers of religion are simply dogmatic. They have no clear idea of God; they only make official proclamations. When one does not understand, he cannot make others understand. But there is no such vanity in Kṛṣṇa consciousness. Kṛṣṇa consciousness is clear in every respect. This is the expected movement Mr. Jung wanted. Every sane man should cooperate with this movement and liberate human society from the gross darkness of ignorance.

Socrates: He Knew Himself—to a Certain Extent

Socrates (470–399 B.C.) turned the attention of his contemporaries toward questions of ethics and virtue. His behavior eventually so angered the authorities in Athens that he was sentenced to death. He could have spared himself by compromising his principles, but he refused and voluntarily drank poison.

Disciple: Socrates strongly opposed the Sophists, a group of speculators who taught that the standards of right and wrong and of truth and falsity were completely relative, being established solely by individual opinion or social convention. Socrates, on the other hand, seemed convinced that there was an absolute, universal truth or good, beyond mere speculation and opinion, that could be known clearly and with certainty.

Śrīla Prabhupāda: He was correct. For our part, since we accept Kṛṣṇa, God, as the supreme authority, the Absolute Truth, we cannot refute what He says. Kṛṣṇa, or God, is by definition supreme perfection, and philosophy is perfect when it is in harmony with Him. This is our position. The philosophy of this Kṛṣṇa consciousness movement is religious in the sense that it is concerned with carrying out the orders of God. That is the sum and substance of religion. It is not possible to manufacture a religion. In the *Śrīmad-Bhāgavatam* manufactured religion is called *kaitava-dharma,* just another form of cheating.

Our basic principle is *dharmaṁ tu sākṣād bhagavat-praṇītam*. The word *dharma* refers to the orders given by God, and if we follow those orders we are following dharma. An individual citizen cannot manufacture laws, for laws are given by the government. Our perfection lies in following the orders of God cent percent. Those who have no conception of God or His orders may manufacture religious systems, but our system is different.

Disciple: The Socratic dialectic usually sought gradually to arrive at an understanding of the essence of a particular moral virtue—for example, self-control, piety, courage, or justice—by examining proposed definitions for completeness and consistency. Socrates wanted to establish more than just a list of universal definitions, however. He tried to show that any particular virtue, when understood in depth, was not different from all the others. The unity of the virtues thus implied the existence of a single absolute good. For Socrates, the goal of life is to rise by means of the intellect to a realization of this absolute good. A person who had attained such knowledge of the good would be self-realized in that he would always do the good without fail. A soul who had thus realized the good was said to be in a healthy or sound state, or to have attained wisdom. Socrates' name for the single absolute good was "knowledge."

Could one say that Socrates was a kind of *jñāna-yogī*?

Śrīla Prabhupāda: Socrates was a *muni,* a great thinker. However, the real truth comes to such a *muni* after many, many births. As Kṛṣṇa says in the *Bhagavad-gītā* [7.19]:

bahūnāṁ janmanām ante jñānavān māṁ prapadyate
vāsudevaḥ sarvam iti sa mahātmā su-durlabhaḥ

"After many births and deaths, he who is actually in knowledge surrenders unto Me, knowing Me to be the cause of all causes and all that is. Such a great soul is very rare."

People like Socrates are known as *jñānavān,* wise men, and after many births they surrender themselves to Kṛṣṇa. They do not do so blindly, but knowing that the Supreme Personality of Godhead is the source of everything. However, this process of self-searching for knowledge takes time. If we take the instructions of Kṛṣṇa directly and surrender unto Him, we save time and many, many births.

Disciple: Socrates terms his method *maieutic,* that is, like that of a midwife. He thought that a soul could not really come to knowledge of the good by the imposition of information from an external source. Rather, such knowledge had to be awakened within the soul itself. The teacher's business is to direct, encourage, and prod a soul until it gives birth to the truth. The *maieutic* method therefore suggests that since the soul is able to bring the truth out of itself, knowledge is really a kind of recollection or remembrance. If so, then there must have been a previous life in which the soul possessed the knowledge it has forgotten. This suggests, then, that the soul (understood as something involving intelligence and memory) exists continuously through many lives and, indeed is eternal.*

Śrīla Prabhupāda: Yes, the soul is eternal. And because the soul is eternal, the intelligence, mind, and senses are also eternal. However, they are all now covered by a material coating, which must be cleansed. Once this material coating is washed away, the real mind, intelligence, and senses will emerge. That is stated in the *Nārada-pañcarātra: tat-paratvena nirmalam.* The purificatory process takes place when one is in touch with the transcendental loving service of the Lord and is chanting the Hare Kṛṣṇa *mahā-mantra.* Caitanya Mahāprabhu said, *ceto-darpaṇa-mārjanam:* one must cleanse the heart. All misconceptions come from misunderstanding. We are all part and parcel of God, yet somehow or other we have forgotten this. Previously our service was rendered to God, but now we are rendering service to something illusory. This is *māyā.* Whether we are liberated or conditioned, our constitutional position is to render service. In the material world we work according to our different capacities—as a politician, a thinker, a poet, or whatever. But if we are disconnected from Kṛṣṇa, all of this is *māyā.* When we perform our duty in order to develop Kṛṣṇa consciousness, our duty enables liberation from this bondage.

Disciple: It is interesting that nowadays we find the kind of relativism taught by Sophists like Protagoras to be again very

*Scholars disagree about whether Socrates explicitly taught the doctrine of remembrance. Even if the doctrine was Plato's, Plato clearly thought it inherent in Socrates' *maieutic* itself.

widespread. "If you believe it, then it is true for you." Socrates took up the task of vigorously combating this position, trying to demonstrate by strong arguments that there must be an absolute truth that is distinguishable from the relative and that must be categorically acknowledged by everyone.

Śrīla Prabhupāda: That is what we are also doing. The Absolute Truth is true for everyone, and the relative truth is relative to a particular position. The relative truth depends on the Absolute Truth, which is the summum bonum. God is the Absolute Truth, and the material world is relative truth. Because the material world is God's energy, it appears to be real or true, just as the reflection of the sun in water emits some light. That reflection is not absolute, and as soon as the sun sets, that light will disappear. Since relative truth is a reflection of the Absolute Truth, the *Śrīmad-Bhāgavatam* states, *satyaṁ paraṁ dhīmahi:* "I worship the Absolute Truth." The Absolute Truth is Kṛṣṇa, Vāsudeva. *Oṁ namo bhagavate vāsudevāya.* This cosmic manifestation is relative truth; it is a manifestation of Kṛṣṇa's external energy. If Kṛṣṇa withdrew His energy, the cosmos would not exist.

In another sense, Kṛṣṇa and Kṛṣṇa's energy are not different. We cannot separate heat from fire; heat is also fire, yet heat is not fire. This is the position of relative truth. As soon as we experience heat, we understand that there is fire. Yet we cannot say that heat is fire. Relative truth is like heat because it stands on the strength of the Absolute Truth, just as heat stands on the strength of fire. Because the Absolute is true, relative truth also appears to be true, although it has no independent existence. A mirage appears to be water because in actuality there is such a thing as water. Similarly, this material world appears attractive because there is actually an all-attractive spiritual world.

Disciple: Socrates held that the highest duty of man was to "care for his soul," that is, to cultivate that healthy state of the soul which is true knowledge, the attainment of the good. When a man becomes fixed in such knowledge he will as a matter of course act correctly in all affairs, he will be beyond the dictates of the passions, and he will remain peaceful and undisturbed in every circumstance. Socrates himself seems to have attained such a state, as his own behavior at the time of his death illustrates: he calmly drank the poison hemlock rather than give up his principles. He seems to have realized knowledge of at least some aspect of the Absolute Truth, although we must add that he never spoke of it as a person or gave it a personal name.

Śrīla Prabhupāda: That is the preliminary stage of understanding the Absolute, known as Brahman realization, realization of the impersonal feature. When one is further advanced he attains Paramātmā realization, realization of the localized feature, whereby he realizes that God is everywhere. It is a fact that God is everywhere, but at the same time God has His own abode. *Goloka eva nivasaty akhilātma-bhūtaḥ.* God is a person, and He has His own abode and associates. Although He is in His abode, He is present everywhere, within every atom (*andāntara-stha-paramāṇu-cayāntara-stham*). Like other impersonalists, Socrates cannot understand how God, through His potency, can remain in His own abode and simultaneously be present in every atom. The material world is His expansion, His energy (*bhūmir āpo 'nalo vāyuḥ khaṁ mano buddhir eva ca*). Because His energy is expanded everywhere, He can be present everywhere. Although the energy and the energetic are nondifferent, we cannot say that they are not distinct. They are simultaneously one and different. This is the perfect philosophy of *acintya-bhedābheda-tattva,* inconceivable simultaneous oneness and difference.

Disciple: Socrates held that "all the virtues are one thing—knowledge." He saw goodness and knowledge as inseparable. This union of the two seems to reflect features of *sattva-guṇa* as described in the *Bhagavad-gītā.*

Śrīla Prabhupāda: *Sattva-guṇa,* the mode of goodness, is a position from which we can receive knowledge. Knowledge cannot be received from the platform of passion and ignorance. If we hear about Kṛṣṇa, or God, we are gradually freed from the clutches of darkness and passion. Then we can come to the platform of *sattva-guṇa,* and when we are perfectly situated there, we are beyond the lower modes. In the words of *Śrīmad-Bhāgavatam* [1.2.18–19]:

naṣṭa-prāyeṣv abhadreṣu nityaṁ bhāgavata-sevayā
bhagavaty uttama-śloke bhaktir bhavati naiṣṭhikī

tadā rajas-tamo-bhāvāḥ kāma-lobhādayaś ca ye
ceta etair anāviddhaṁ sthitaṁ sattve prasīdati

"For one who regularly attends classes on the *Śrīmad-Bhāgavatam* and renders service to the pure devotee, all that is troublesome to the heart is almost completely destroyed, and loving service unto the Personality of Godhead, who is praised with transcendental songs, is established as an irrevocable fact. As soon as irrevocable loving service is established in the heart, the effects of nature's modes of passion and ignorance, such as lust, desire, and hankering, disappear from the heart. Then the devotee is established in goodness, and he becomes completely happy."

This process may be gradual, but it is certain. The more we hear about Kṛṣṇa, the more we become purified. Purification means freedom from the attacks of greed and passion. Then we can become happy. From the *brahma-bhūta* platform we can realize ourselves and then realize God. So before realizing the Supreme Good, we must first come to the platform of *sattva-guṇa,* goodness. Therefore we have regulations prohibiting illicit sex, meat-eating, intoxication, and gambling. Ultimately we must transcend even the mode of goodness through *bhakti.* Then we become liberated, gradually develop love of God, and regain our original state. *Muktir hitvānyathā rūpam svarūpeṇa vyavasthitiḥ.* This means giving up all material engagements and rendering full service to Kṛṣṇa. Then we attain the state where *māyā* cannot touch us. If we keep in touch with Kṛṣṇa, *māyā* has no jurisdiction.

Māyām etāṁ taranti te. This is perfection.

Disciple: Socrates took the oracular *gnothi seauton,* "know thyself," to enjoin "care of the soul." Care of the soul, as we have seen, involved an intense intellectual endeavor, a kind of introspective contemplation or meditation. It gradually purified the self, detaching it more and more from the body and its passions. Thus through the contemplative endeavor entailed by "know thyself," a person attained knowledge and self-control, and with that he also became happy.

Śrīla Prabhupāda: Yes, that is a fact. Meditation means analyzing the self and searching for the Absolute Truth. That is described in the Vedic literatures: *dhyānāvasthita-tad-gatena manasā paśyanti yaṁ yoginaḥ.* Through meditation, the yogi sees the Supreme Truth (Kṛṣṇa, or God) within himself. Kṛṣṇa is there. The yogi consults with Kṛṣṇa, and Kṛṣṇa advises him. That is the relationship Kṛṣṇa has with the yogi. *Dadāmi buddhi-yogaṁ tam.* When one is purified, he is always seeing Kṛṣṇa within himself. This is confirmed in the *Brahma-saṁhitā* [5.38]:

premāñjana-cchurita-bhakti-vilocanena
santaḥ sadaiva hṛdayeṣu vilokayanti
yaṁ śyāmasundaram acintya-guṇa-svarūpaṁ
govindam ādi-puruṣaṁ tam ahaṁ bhajāmi

"I worship the primeval Lord, Govinda, who is always seen by the devotee whose eyes are anointed with the pulp of love. He is seen in His eternal form of Śyāmasundara, situated within the heart of the devotee." Thus an advanced saintly person is always seeing Kṛṣṇa. In this verse, the word *śyāmasundara* means "blackish but at the same time extraordinarily beautiful." Being the Supreme Personality of Godhead, Kṛṣṇa is of course very beautiful. The word *acintya* means that He has inconceivable, unlimited qualities. Although He is situated everywhere, as Govinda He is always dancing in Vṛndāvana with the *gopīs.* There He plays with His friends and sometimes, acting as a naughty boy, teases

His mother. These pastimes of the Supreme Person are described in the *Śrīmad-Bhāgavatam.*

Disciple: As far as we know, Socrates himself had no teacher in philosophy. Indeed, he refers to himself as "self-made." Do you believe that one can be self-taught? Can self-knowledge be attained through one's own meditation or introspection?

Śrīla Prabhupāda: Yes. Ordinarily everyone thinks according to the bodily conception. If I begin to study the different parts of my body and seriously begin to consider what I am, I will gradually arrive at the study of the soul. If I ask myself, "Am I this hand?" the answer will be "No, I am not this hand. Rather, this is my hand." I can thus continue analyzing each part of the body and discover that all the parts are mine but that I am different. Through this method of self-study, any intelligent man can see that he is not the body. This is the first lesson of the *Bhagavad-gītā* [2.13]:

dehino 'smin yathā dehe kaumāraṁ yauvanaṁ jarā
tathā dehāntara-prāptir dhīras tatra na muhyati

"As the embodied soul continuously passes, in this body, from boyhood to youth to old age, the soul similarly passes into another body at death. A sober person is not bewildered by such a change."

At one time I had the body of a child, but now that body is no longer existing. Nonetheless, I am aware that I possessed such a body; therefore from this I can deduce that I am something other than the body. I may rent an apartment, but I do not identify with it. The body may be mine, but I am not the body. By this kind of introspection, a man can teach himself the distinction between the body and the soul.

As far as being *completely* self-taught, according to the *Bhagavad-gītā* and the Vedic conception, life is continuous. Since we are always acquiring experience, we cannot actually say that Socrates was self-taught. Rather, in his previous lives he had cultivated knowledge, and this knowledge was simply continuing. That is a fact. Otherwise, why is one man intelligent and another man ignorant? This is due to continuity.

Disciple: Socrates believed that through intellectual endeavor—meditation—a person can attain knowledge or wisdom, which is nothing else but the possession of all the virtues in their unity. Such a person always acts in the right way and thus is happy. Therefore the enlightened man is meditative, knowledgeable, and virtuous. He is also happy because he acts properly.

Śrīla Prabhupāda: Yes, that is confirmed in the *Bhagavad-gītā* [18.54]. *Brahma-bhūtaḥ prasannātmā na śocati na kāṅkṣati:* when one is self-realized, he immediately becomes happy, joyful (*prasannātmā).* This is because he is properly situated. One may labor a long time under some mistaken idea, but when he finally comes to the proper conclusion, he becomes very happy. He thinks, "Oh, what a fool I was, going on so long in such a mistaken way." Thus a self-realized person is happy.

Happiness means that one no longer has to think of attaining things. For instance, Dhruva Mahārāja told the Lord, *svāmin kṛtārtho 'smi varaṁ na yāce:* "Having seen You, my Lord, I don't want any material benediction." Prahlāda Mahārāja also said, "My Lord, I don't want material benefits. I have seen my father—who was such a big materialist that even the demigods were afraid of him—destroyed by You within a second. Therefore I am not after these things."

So real knowledge means that one no longer hankers for anything. The *karmīs* [fruitive workers], *jñānīs* [speculators], and yogis are all hankering after something. The *karmīs* want material wealth, beautiful women, and good positions. If one is not hankering for what one does not have, he is lamenting for what he has lost. The *jñānīs* are also hankering, expecting to become one with God and merge into His existence. And the yogis are hankering after some magical powers to befool others into thinking that they have become God. In India some yogis convince people that they can manufacture gold and fly in the sky, and foolish people believe them. Even if a yogi can fly, what is his great achievement? There are many birds flying. What is the difference? An intelligent person can understand this. If a person says that he will walk on water, thousands of fools will come to see him. People will even pay ten rupees just to see a man bark like a dog, not thinking that there are many dogs barking anyway. In any case, people are always hankering and lamenting, but the devotee is fully satisfied in the service of the Lord. He doesn't hanker for anything, nor does he lament.

Disciple: Through *jñāna,* philosophical inquiry, could Socrates have realized Brahman?

Śrīla Prabhupāda: Yes.

Disciple: But what about the realization of Bhagavān, Kṛṣṇa? I thought that Kṛṣṇa can be realized only through *bhakti,* devotion.

Śrīla Prabhupāda: Yes, one cannot enter into Kṛṣṇa's abode without being a purified *bhakta* [devotee]. Kṛṣṇa states that in the *Bhagavad-gītā* [18.55]. *Bhaktyā mām abhijānāti:* "One can understand Me as I am only by devotional service." Kṛṣṇa never says that He can be understood by *jñāna, karma,* or yoga. The personal abode of Kṛṣṇa is especially reserved for the *bhaktas,* and the *jñānīs,* yogis, and *karmīs* cannot go there.

Disciple: What do you mean when you say that Kṛṣṇa consciousness is the ultimate goal of life? Does this mean always being conscious of Kṛṣṇa?

Śrīla Prabhupāda: Yes, we should always be thinking of Kṛṣṇa. We should act in such a way that we have to think of Kṛṣṇa all the time. For instance, we are discussing Socratic philosophy in order to strengthen our Kṛṣṇa consciousness. Therefore the ultimate goal is Kṛṣṇa; otherwise we are not interested in criticizing or accepting anyone's philosophy. We are neutral.

Disciple: So the proper use of intelligence is to guide everything in such a way that we become Kṛṣṇa conscious?

Śrīla Prabhupāda: That's it. Without Kṛṣṇa consciousness, we remain on the mental platform. Being on the mental platform means hovering. On that platform, we are not fixed. It is the business of the mind to accept this and reject that, but when we are fixed in Kṛṣṇa consciousness we are no longer subjected to the mind's acceptance or rejection.

Disciple: Right conduct then becomes automatic?

Śrīla Prabhupāda: Yes, as soon as the mind wanders, we should immediately drag it back to concentrate on Kṛṣṇa. While chanting, our mind sometimes wanders far away, but when we become conscious of this, we should immediately bring the mind back to hear the sound vibration of "Hare Kṛṣṇa." That is called *yoga-abhyāsa,* the practice of *yoga.* We should not allow our mind to wander elsewhere. We should simply chant and hear the Hare Kṛṣṇa *mantra,* for that is the best *yoga* system.

Disciple: Socrates could have avoided the death penalty if he had compromised his convictions. He refused to do this and so became a martyr for his beliefs.

Śrīla Prabhupāda: It is good that he stuck to his point yet regrettable that he lived in a society in which he could not think independently. Therefore he was obliged to die. In that sense, Socrates was a great soul because although he appeared in a society that was not very advanced, he was still such a great philosopher.

Origen: The Original Christian Mystic

An influential founder of the Christian Church, Origen of Alexandria (A.D. circa 185–circa 254) ranks among its most prolific writers. Known as the father of Christian mysticism, he taught reincarnation—and was martyred for it.

Disciple: Origen is generally considered the founder of formal Christian philosophy, because he was the first to attempt to establish Christianity on the basis of philosophy as well as faith. He believed that the ultimate spiritual reality consists of the supreme, infinite person, God, as well as individual personalities. Ultimate reality may be defined as the relationships of persons with one another and with the infinite person Himself. In this view, Origen differs from the Greeks, who were basically impersonalists.

Śrīla Prabhupāda: Our Vedic conception is almost the same. Individual souls, which we call living entities, are always present, and each one of them has an intimate relationship with the Supreme Personality of Godhead. In material, conditioned life, the living entity has forgotten this relationship. By rendering devotional service, he attains the liberated position and at that time revives his relationship with the Supreme Personality of Godhead.

Disciple: Origen ascribed to a doctrine of the Trinity, in which God the Father is supreme. God the Son, called the *Logos,* is subordinate to the Father. It is the Son who brings the material world into existence. That is, God the Father is not the direct creator; rather, it is the Son who creates directly, like Lord Brahmā. The third aspect of the Trinity is the Holy Spirit, who is subordinate to the Son. According to Origen, all three of these aspects are divine and co-eternal. They have always existed simultaneously as the Trinity of God.

Śrīla Prabhupāda: According to the *Vedas,* Kṛṣṇa is the original Personality of Godhead. As He confirms in the

Bhagavad-gītā: ahaṁ sarvasya prabhavaḥ. "I am the source of all spiritual and material worlds" [*Bhagavad-gītā* 10.8]. Whether you call this origin the Father or the Holy Spirit, it doesn't matter. The Supreme Personality of Godhead is the origin. According to the Vedic conception, there are two types of expansions: God's personal expansions, called *viṣṇu-tattva,* and His partial part-and-parcel expansions, called *jīva-tattva.* There are many varieties of personal expansions: *puruṣa-avatāras, manvantara-avatāras,* and so on. For the creation of this material world, the Lord expands as Brahmā, Viṣṇu, and Maheśvara [Śiva]. Viṣṇu is a personal expansion, and Brahmā is a *jīva-tattva* expansion. Between the personal *viṣṇu-tattva* expansions and the *jīva-tattva* expansions is a kind of intermediate expansion called Śiva, or Maheśvara. The material ingredients are given, and Brahmā creates each universe. Viṣṇu maintains the creation, and Lord Śiva annihilates it. It is the nature of the external potency to be created, maintained, and dissolved. More detailed information is given in the *Caitanya-caritāmṛta.*

In any case, the *jīvas,* or living entities, are all considered sons of God. They are situated in one of two positions: liberated or conditioned. Those who are liberated can personally associate with the Supreme Personality of Godhead, and those who are conditioned within this material world have forgotten the Supreme Lord. Therefore they suffer within this material world in different bodily forms. They can be elevated, however, through the practice of Kṛṣṇa consciousness under the guidance of the *śāstras* [scriptures] and the bona fide guru.

Disciple: Origen believed that it is through the combined working of divine grace and man's free will that the individual soul attains perfection, which consists of attaining a personal relationship with the infinite Person.

Śrīla Prabhupāda: Yes, and that is called *bhakti-mārga,* the path of devotional service to the Supreme Personality of Godhead, Bhagavān. The Absolute Truth is manifested in three features: Brahman, Paramātmā, and Bhagavān.

Bhagavān is the personal feature, and the Paramātmā, situated in everyone's heart, may be compared to the Holy Spirit. The Brahman feature is present everywhere. The highest perfection of spiritual life includes the understanding of the personal feature of the Lord. When one understands Bhagavān, one engages in His service. In this way, the living entity is situated in his original constitutional position and is eternally blissful.

Disciple: Origen considered that just as man's free will precipitated his fall, man's free will can also bring about his salvation. Man can return to God by practicing material detachment. Such detachment can be made possible by help from the *Logos,* the Christ.

Śrīla Prabhupāda: Yes, that is also our conception. The fallen soul is transmigrating within this material world, up and down in different forms of life. When his consciousness is sufficiently developed, he can be enlightened by God, who gives him instructions in the *Bhagavad-gītā.* Through the spiritual master's help, he can attain full enlightenment. When he understands his transcendental position of bliss, he automatically gives up material bodily attachments. Then he attains freedom. The living entity attains his normal, constitutional position when he is properly situated in his spiritual identity and engaged in the service of the Lord.

Disciple: Origen believed that all the elements found in the material body are also found in the spiritual body, which he called the "interior man." Origen writes: "There are two men in each of us. . . . As every exterior man has for homonym the interior man, so it is for all his members, and one can say that every member of the exterior man can be found under this name in the interior man." Thus for every sense that we possess in the exterior body, there is a corresponding sense in the interior body, or spiritual body.

Śrīla Prabhupāda: The spirit soul is now within this material body, but originally the spirit soul had no material body. The spiritual body of the spirit soul is eternally existing. The material body is simply a coating of the spiritual body. The material body is cut, like a suit, according to the spiritual body. The material elements—earth, water, air, fire, etc.—become like clay when mixed together, and they coat the spiritual body. It is because the spiritual body has a shape that the material body also takes a shape. In actuality, the material body has nothing to do with the spiritual body; it is but a kind of contamination causing the suffering of the spirit soul. As soon as the spirit soul is coated with this material contamination, he identifies himself with the coating and forgets his real spiritual body. That is called *māyā,* ignorance or illusion. This ignorance continues as long as we are not fully Kṛṣṇa conscious. When we become fully Kṛṣṇa conscious, we understand that the material body is but the external coating and that we are different. When we attain this uncontaminated understanding, we arrive at what is called the *brahma-bhūta* platform. When the spirit soul, which is Brahman, is under the illusion of the material bodily conditioning, we are on the *jīva-bhūta* platform. *Brahma-bhūta* is attained when we no longer identify with the material body but with the spirit soul within. When we come to this platform, we become joyful.

brahma-bhūtaḥ prasannātmā na śocati na kāṅkṣati
samaḥ sarveṣu bhūteṣu mad-bhaktiṁ labhate parām

"One who is thus transcendentally situated at once realizes the Supreme Brahman and becomes fully joyful. He never laments or desires to have anything. He is equally disposed toward every living entity. In that state he attains pure devotional service unto Me" [*Bhagavad-gītā* 18.54]. In this position one sees all living entities as spirit souls; he does not see the outward covering. When he sees a dog, he sees a spirit soul covered by the body of a dog. This state is also described in the *Bhagavad-gītā.*

vidyā-vinaya-sampanne brāhmaṇe gavi hastini
śuni caiva śva-pāke ca paṇḍitāḥ sama-darśinaḥ

"The humble sages, by virtue of true knowledge, see with equal vision a learned and gentle *brāhmaṇa,* a cow, an elephant, a dog and a dog-eater [outcaste]" [*Bhagavad-gītā* 5.18]. When one is in the body of an animal, he cannot understand his spiritual identity. This identity can best be realized in a human civilization in which the *varṇāśrama* system is practiced. This system divides life into four *āśramas* (*brāhmaṇa, kṣatriya, vaiśya,* and *śūdra*) and four *varṇas* (*brahmacārī, gṛhastha, vānaprastha,* and *sannyāsa*). The highest position is that of a *brāhmaṇa-sannyāsī,* a platform from which one may best realize his original constitutional position, act accordingly, and thus attain deliverance, or *mukti. Mukti* means understanding our constitutional position and acting accordingly. Conditioned life, a life of bondage, means identifying with the body and acting on the bodily platform. On the *mukti* platform, our activities differ from those enacted on the conditioned platform. Devotional service is rendered from the *mukti* platform. If we engage in devotional service, we maintain our spiritual identity and are therefore liberated, even though inhabiting the conditioned, material body.

Disciple: Origen also believed that the interior man, or the spiritual body, also has spiritual senses that enable the soul to taste, see, touch, and contemplate the things of God.

Śrīla Prabhupāda: Yes. That is devotional life.

Disciple: During his lifetime, Origen was a famous teacher and was very much in demand. For him, teaching meant explaining the words of God and no more. He believed that a preacher must first be a man of prayer and must be in contact with God. He should not pray for material goods but for a better understanding of the scriptures.

Śrīla Prabhupāda: Yes, that is a real preacher. As explained in Vedic literatures: *śravaṇaṁ kīrtanam,* First of all, we become perfect by hearing. This is called *śravaṇam.* When we are thus situated by hearing perfectly from an authorized person, our next stage begins: *kīrtanam,* preaching. In this material world, everyone is hearing something from someone else. In order to pass examinations, a student must hear his professor. Then, in his own right, he can become a professor himself. If we hear from a bona fide spiritual master, we become perfect and can become real preachers. We should preach about Kṛṣṇa for Kṛṣṇa, not for any person within this material world. We should hear and preach about the Supreme Person, the transcendental Personality of Godhead. That is the duty of a liberated soul.

Disciple: As far as contradictions and seeming absurdities in scripture are concerned, Origen considered them to be stumbling blocks permitted to exist by God in order for man to pass beyond the literal meaning. He writes that "everything in scripture has a spiritual meaning, but not all of it has a literal meaning."

Śrīla Prabhupāda: Generally speaking, every word in scripture has a literal meaning, but people cannot understand it properly because they do not hear from the proper person. They interpret instead. There is no need to interpret the words of God. Sometimes the words of God cannot be understood by an ordinary person; therefore we may require the transparent medium of the guru. Since the guru is fully cognizant of the words spoken by God, we are advised to receive the words of the scriptures through the guru. There is no ambiguity in the words of God, but due to our imperfect knowledge, we sometimes cannot understand. Not understanding, we try to interpret, but because we are imperfect, our interpretations are also imperfect. The conclusion is that the words of God, the scriptures, should be understood from a person who has realized God.

Disciple: Origen did not believe that the individual soul has been existing from all eternity. It was created. He writes: "The rational natures that were made in the beginning did not always exist; they came into being when they were created."

Śrīla Prabhupāda: That is not correct. Both the living entity and God are simultaneously eternally existing, and the living entity is part and parcel of God. Although eternally existing, the living entity is changing his body. *Na hanyate hanyamāne śarīre* [*Bhagavad-gītā* 2.20]. One body after another is being created and destroyed, but the living being himself exists eternally. So we disagree when Origen says that the soul is created. Our spiritual identity is never created. That is the difference between spirit and matter. Material things are created, but spirit is without beginning.

na tv evāhaṁ jātu nāsaṁ na tvaṁ neme janādhipāḥ
na caiva na bhaviṣyāmaḥ sarve vayam ataḥ param

"Never was there a time when I did not exist, nor you, nor all these kings; nor in the future shall any of us cease to be" [*Bhagavad-gītā* 2.12].

Disciple: Origen differed from later Church doctrine in his belief in transmigration. Although he believed that the soul was originally created, he also believed that it transmigrated because it could always refuse to give itself to God. So he saw the individual soul as possibly rising and falling perpetually on the evolutionary scale. Later Church doctrine held that one's choice for eternity is made in this one lifetime. As Origen saw it, the individual soul, falling short of the ultimate goal, is reincarnated again and again.

Śrīla Prabhupāda: Yes, that is the Vedic version. Unless one is liberated and goes to the kingdom of God, he must transmigrate from one material body to another. The material body grows, remains for some time, reproduces, grows old, and becomes useless. Then the living entity has to leave one body for another. Once in a new body, he again attempts to fulfill his desires, and again he goes through the process of dying and accepting another material body. This is the process of transmigration.

Disciple: It is interesting that neither Origen nor Christ rejected transmigration. It wasn't until Augustine that it was denied.

Śrīla Prabhupāda: Transmigration is a fact. A person cannot wear the same clothes all of his life. Our clothes become old and useless, and we have to change them. The living being is certainly eternal, but he has to accept a material body for material sense gratification, and such a body cannot endure perpetually, just as our clothes cannot last forever. All of this is thoroughly explained in the *Bhagavad-gītā:*

dehino 'smin yathā dehe kaumāraṁ yauvanaṁ jarā
tathā dehāntara-prāptir dhīras tatra na muhyati

"As the embodied soul continuously passes, in this body, from boyhood to youth to old age, the soul similarly passes into another body at death. A sober person is not bewildered by such a change" [*Bhagavad-gītā* 2.13].

śarīraṁ yad avāpnoti yac cāpy utkrāmatīśvaraḥ
gṛhītvaitāni saṁyāti vāyur gandhān ivāśayāt

"The living entity in the material world carries his different conceptions of life from one body to another as the air carries aromas. Thus he takes one kind of body and again quits it to take another" [*Bhagavad-gītā* 15.8].

So, this proces of transmigration will continue until one attains liberation and goes back home, back to Godhead.

Thomas Aquinas: In Search of Divine Essence

Thomas Aquinas (1225?–1274) was the leading Christian philosopher of the middle ages. He led an austere life as a celibate monk, writing prolifically and teaching widely.

Disciple: Thomas Aquinas compiled the entire Church doctrine in *Summa Theologiae,* which constitutes the official philosophy of the Roman Catholic Church. Aquinas did not make Augustine's sharp distinction between the material and spiritual worlds, or between secular society and the city of God. For him, both material and spiritual creations have their origin in God. At the same time, he admits that the spiritual world is superior to the material.

Śrīla Prabhupāda: When we speak of "material world," we refer to that which is temporary. Some philosophers, like the Māyāvādīs [impersonalists], claim that the material world is false, but we Vaiṣṇavas prefer to say that it is temporary or illusory. It is a reflection of the spiritual world, but in itself it has no reality. We therefore sometimes compare the material world to a mirage in the desert. In the material world there is no happiness, but the transcendental bliss and happiness existing in the spiritual world are reflected here. Unintelligent people chase after this illusory happiness, forgetting the real happiness that is in spiritual life.

Disciple: Aquinas agreed with both the statements of Anselm and Abelard: "I believe in order that I may understand," and, "I understand in order that I may believe." Thus reason and revelation complement one another as a means to truth.

Śrīla Prabhupāda: Since human reason is not perfect, revelation is also needed. The truth is attained through logic, philosophy, and revelation. According to the Vaiṣṇava tradition, we arrive at the truth through the guru, the spiritual master, who is accepted as the representative of the Absolute Truth, the Personality of Godhead. He transmits the message of the truth because he has seen the Absolute Truth through the disciplic succession. If we accept the bona fide spiritual master and please him by submissive service, by virtue of his mercy and pleasure we can understand God and the spiritual world by revelation. We therefore offer our respects to the spiritual master in the prayer:

yasya prasādād bhagavat-prasādo
yasyāprasādān na gatiḥ kuto 'pi
dhyāyan stuvaṁs tasya yaśas tri-sandhyaṁ
vande guroḥ śrī-caraṇāravindam

"By the mercy of the spiritual master one receives the benediction of Kṛṣṇa. Without the grace of the spiritual master, one cannot make any advancement. Therefore, I should always remember and praise the spiritual master, offering respectful obeisances unto his lotus feet at least three times a day" [*Śrī Gurv-aṣṭaka* 8]. We can understand God if we please the spiritual master, who carries the Lord's message without speculation. It is stated in the *Padma Purāṇa: sevonmukhe hi jihvādau svayam eva sphuraty adaḥ*. When we engage our senses in the Lord's service, the Lord is revealed.

Disciple: For Aquinas, God is the only single essence that consists of pure form. He felt that matter is only a potential and, in order to be real, must assume a certain shape or form. In other words, the living entity has to acquire an individual form in order to actualize himself. When matter unites with form, the form gives individuality and personality.

Śrīla Prabhupāda: Matter in itself has no form; it is the spirit soul that has form. Matter is a covering for the actual form of the spirit soul. Because the soul has form, matter appears to have form. Matter is like cloth that is cut to fit the body. In the spiritual world, however, everything has form: God and the spirit souls.

Disciple: Aquinas believed that only God and the angels have nonmaterial form. There is no difference between

God's form and God's spiritual Self.
Śrīla Prabhupāda: Both the individual souls and God have form. That is real form. Material form is but a covering for the spiritual body.
Disciple: Aquinas set forth five basic arguments for God's existence: first, God necessarily exists as the first cause; second, the material world cannot create itself but needs something external, or spiritual, to create it; third, because the world exists, there must be a creator; fourth, since there is relative perfection in the world, there must be absolute perfection underlying it; and fifth, since the creation has design and purpose, there must be a designer who planned it.
Śrīla Prabhupāda: We also honor these arguments. Also, without a father and mother, children cannot be brought into existence. Modern philosophers do not consider this strongest argument. According to the *Brahma-saṁhitā,* everything has a cause, and God is the ultimate cause.

īśvaraḥ paramaḥ kṛṣṇaḥ sac-cid-ānanda-vigrahaḥ
anādir ādir govindaḥ sarva-kāraṇa-kāraṇam

"Kṛṣṇa, who is known as Govinda, is the supreme controller. He has an eternal, blissful, spiritual body. He is the origin of all. He has no other origin, for He is the prime cause of all causes" [*Brahma-saṁhitā* 5.1].
Disciple: He also states that the relative perfection we find here necessitates an absolute perfection.
Śrīla Prabhupāda: Yes, the spiritual world is absolute perfection, and this temporary material world is but a reflection of that spiritual world. Whatever perfection we find in this material world is derived from the spiritual world. *Janmādy asya yataḥ.* According to the *Vedānta-sūtra,* whatever is generated comes from the Absolute Truth.
Disciple: Today, some scientists even admit Aquinas's argument that since nothing can create itself in this material world, something external, or spiritual, is required for initial creation.

Śrīla Prabhupāda: Yes, a mountain cannot create anything, but a human being can give form to a stone. A mountain may be very large, but it remains a stone incapable of giving shape to anything.
Disciple: Unlike Plato and Aristotle, Aquinas maintained that God created the universe out of nothing.
Śrīla Prabhupāda: No, the universe is created by God, certainly, but God and His energies are always there. You cannot logically say that the universe was created out of nothing.
Disciple: Aquinas would contend that since the material universe could not have arisen out of God's spiritual nature, it had to be created out of nothing.
Śrīla Prabhupāda: Material nature is also an energy of God's. As Kṛṣṇa states in the *Bhagavad-gītā:*

bhūmir āpo 'nalo vāyuḥ khaṁ mano buddhir eva ca
ahaṅkāra itīyaṁ me bhinnā prakṛtir aṣṭadhā

"Earth, water, fire, air, ether, mind, intelligence, and false ego—all together these eight constitute My separated material energies" [*Bhagavad-gītā* 7.4]. All of these energies emanate from God, and therefore they are not unreal. They are considered inferior because they are God's separated material energies. The sound that comes from a tape recorder may sound exactly like the original person's voice. The sound is not the person's voice itself, but it has come from the person. If one cannot see where the sound is coming from, one may suppose that the person is actually speaking, although he may be far away. Similarly, the material world is an expansion of the Supreme Lord's energy, and we should not think that it has been brought into existence out of nothing. It has emanated from the Supreme Truth, but it is the inferior, separated energy. The superior energy is found in the spiritual world, which is the world of reality. In any case we cannot agree that the material world has come from nothing.
Disciple: Well, Aquinas would say that it was created by God out of nothing.

Śrīla Prabhupāda: You cannot say that God's energy is nothing. His energy is exhibited and is eternally existing with Him. God's energy must be there. If God doesn't have energy, how can He be God?

na tasya kāryaṁ karaṇaṁ ca vidyate
na tat-samaś cābhyadhikaś ca dṛśyate
parāsya śaktir vividhaiva śrūyate
svābhāvikī jñāna-bala-kriyā ca

"The Supreme Lord has no duty to perform, and no one is found to be equal to or greater than Him, for everything is done naturally and systematically by His multifarious energies" [*Śvetāśvatara Upaniṣad* 6.8]. God has multi-energies, and the material energy is but one. Since God is everything, you cannot say that the material universe comes from nothing.

Disciple: Like Augustine, Aquinas believed that sin and man are concomitant. Due to Adam's original sin, all men require salvation, which can be obtained only through God's grace. But the individual has to assent by his free will for God's grace to function.

Śrīla Prabhupāda: Yes, we call that assent *bhakti,* devotional service.

ataḥ śrī-kṛṣṇa-nāmādi na bhaved grāhyam indriyaiḥ
sevonmukhe hi jihvādau svayam eva sphuraty adaḥ

"Material senses cannot appreciate Kṛṣṇa's holy name, form, qualities, and pastimes. When a conditioned soul is awakened to Kṛṣṇa consciousness and renders service by using his tongue to chant the Lord's holy name and to taste the remnants of His food, the soul's consciousness becomes purified, and gradually Kṛṣṇa reveals who He really is" [*Padma Purāṇa*].

Bhakti is our eternal engagement, and when we engage in our eternal activities, we attain salvation, or liberation. When we engage in false activities, we are in illusion, *māyā*. *Mukti,* liberation, means remaining in our constitutional position. In the material world, we engage in many different activities, but they all refer to the material body. In the spiritual world, the spirit engages in the Lord's service, and this is liberation, or salvation.

Disciple: Aquinas considered sins to be both venial and mortal. A venial sin is one that can be pardoned, but a mortal sin cannot. A mortal sin stains the soul.

Śrīla Prabhupāda: When a living entity disobeys the orders of God, he is put into this material world, and that is his punishment. He either rectifies himself by good association or undergoes transmigration. By taking on one body after another, he is subject to the tribulations of material existence. The soul is not stained, but he can participate in sinful activity. As soon as we are in contact with the material nature, we come under the clutches of the material world.

prakṛteḥ kriyamāṇāni guṇaiḥ karmāṇi sarvaśaḥ
ahaṅkāra-vimūḍhātmā kartāham iti manyate

"The spirit soul bewildered by the influence of false ego thinks himself the doer of activities that are in actuality carried out by the three modes of material nature" [*Bhagavad-gītā* 3.27]. As soon as the living entity enters the material world, he loses his own power. He is completely under the clutches of material nature. Oil never mixes with water, but it may be carried away by the waves.

Disciple: Aquinas felt that the monastic vows of poverty, celibacy, and obedience give a direct path to God, but he did not think that these austerities were meant for the masses of men. He looked on life as a pilgrimage through the world of the senses to the spiritual world of God, from imperfection to perfection, and the monastic vows are meant to help us on this path.

Śrīla Prabhupāda: Yes, according to the Vedic instructions, we must take to the path of *tapasya,* voluntary self-denial.

Tapasā brahmacaryeṇa. Tapasya, or austerity, begins with *brahmacarya,* celibacy. We must first learn to control the sex urge. That is the beginning of *tapasya.* We must control the senses and the mind, and then we should give everything that we have to the Lord's service. By following the path of truth and remaining clean, we can practice yoga. In this way, it is possible to advance toward the spiritual kingdom.

All of this can be realized, however, by engaging in devotional service. If we become devotees of Kṛṣṇa, we automatically attain the benefits of austerities without having to make a separate effort. By one stroke, devotional service, we can acquire the benefits of all the other processes.

Disciple: Aquinas did not believe in a soul per se as being divorced from a particular form. God did not create a soul capable of inhabiting any body or form; rather, He created an angelic soul, a human soul, and an animal soul, or a plant soul. Here again, we find the conception of the soul's creation.

Śrīla Prabhupāda: The soul is not created but is eternally existing along with God. The soul has the independence to turn from God, in which case he becomes like a spark falling from a great fire. When the spark is separated, it loses its illumination. In any case, the individual soul is always there. The master and His servants are there eternally. We cannot say that the parts of a body are separately created. As soon as the body is present, all the parts are there with it. The soul is never created, and it never dies. This is confirmed in the very beginning of the *Bhagavad-gītā:*

na jāyate mriyate vā kadācin
nāyaṁ bhūtvā bhavitā vā na bhūyaḥ
ajo nityaḥ śāśvato 'yaṁ purāṇo
na hanyate hanyamāne śarīre

"For the soul there is neither birth nor death at any time. He has not come into being, does not come into being, and will not come into being. He is unborn, eternal, ever-existing, and primeval. He is not slain when the body is slain" [*Bhagavad-gītā* 2.20]. It may appear that the soul comes into existence and dies, but this is because he has accepted the material body. When the soul is liberated, he doesn't have to accept another material body. He can return home, back to Godhead, in his original spiritual body.

The soul was never created but is always existing with God. If we say that the soul was created, the question may be raised whether or not God, the Supreme Soul, was also created. Of course, this is not the case. God is eternal, and His parts and parcels are also eternal. The difference is that God never accepts a material body, whereas the individual soul, being but a small particle, sometimes succumbs to the material energy.

Disciple: Is the soul eternally existing with God in a spiritual form?

Śrīla Prabhupāda: Yes.

Disciple: So the soul has a form that is incorruptible. Is this not also the form of the material body?

Śrīla Prabhupāda: The material body is an imitation. It is false. Because the spiritual body has form, the material body, which is a coating, takes on form. As I have already explained, a cloth originally has no form, but a tailor can cut the cloth to fit a form. In actuality, this material form is illusory. The elements of this material form originally have no form. They take on form for a while, and when the body becomes old and useless, they return to their original position. In the *Bhagavad-gītā* [18.61] the body is compared to a machine. The soul has his own form, but he is given a machine, the body, which he uses to wander throughout the universe, attempting to enjoy himself.

Disciple: Aquinas considered that sex is meant exclusively for the begetting of children, and that the parents are responsible for giving their children a spiritual education.

Śrīla Prabhupāda: That is also the Vedic injunction. You should not beget children unless you can liberate them from the cycle of birth and death.

gurur na sa syāt sva-jano na sa syāt
pitā na sa syāj jananī na sā syāt
daivaṁ na tat syān na patiś ca sa syān
na mocayed yaḥ samupeta-mṛtyum

"One who cannot deliver his dependents from the path of repeated birth and death should never become a spiritual master, a father, a husband, a mother, or a worshipable demigod" [*Śrīmad-Bhāgavatam* 5.5.18].

Disciple: Aquinas argued that sex for reasons other than propagation is "repugnant of the good of nature, which is the conservation of the species." Considering today's overpopulation, does this argument still hold?

Śrīla Prabhupāda: The conservation of the species doesn't enter into it. Illicit sex is sinful because it is for sense gratification instead of for begetting children. Sense gratification in any form is sinful.

Disciple: Concerning the state, Aquinas, like Plato, believed in an enlightened monarchy, but in certain cases he felt it is not necessary for man to obey human laws if they are opposed to human welfare and are instruments of violence.

Śrīla Prabhupāda: Yes, but first of all we must know what our welfare is. Unfortunately, as materialistic education advances, we are missing the aim of life. Life's aim is declared openly in the *Vedānta-sūtra: athāto brahma-jijñāsā.* Life is meant for understanding the Absolute Truth. Vedic civilization is based on this principle, but modern civilization has deviated and is devoting itself to that which cannot possibly relieve us from the tribulations of birth, old age, disease, and death. So-called scientific advancement has not solved life's real problems. Although we are eternal, we are presently subjected to birth and death. In this age of quarrel (Kali-yuga), people are slow to learn about self-realization. People create their own way of life, and they are unfortunate and disturbed.

Disciple: Aquinas concludes that if the laws of God and man conflict, we should obey the laws of God.

Śrīla Prabhupāda: Yes. We can also obey the man who obeys the laws of God. It is useless to obey an imperfect person. That is the blind following the blind. If the leader does not follow the instructions of the supreme controller, he is necessarily blind, and he cannot lead. Why should we risk our lives by following blind men who believe that they are knowledgeable but are not? We should instead decide to take lessons from the Supreme Person, Kṛṣṇa, who knows everything perfectly. Kṛṣṇa knows past, present, and future, and what is for our benefit.

Disciple: For Aquinas, all earthly powers exist only by God's permission. Since the Church is God's emissary on earth, the Church should control secular power as well. He felt that secular rulers should remain subservient to the Church, which should be able to excommunicate a monarch and dethrone him.

Śrīla Prabhupāda: World activities should be regulated so that God is the ultimate goal of understanding. Although the Church, or the *brāhmaṇas,* may not directly carry out administrative activities, the government should function under their supervision and instructions. That is the Vedic system. The administrators, the *kṣatriyas,* used to take instructions from the *brāhmaṇas,* who could deliver a spiritual message. It is mentioned in the *Bhagavad-gītā* [4.1] that millions of years ago Kṛṣṇa instructed the sun-god in the yoga of the *Bhagavad-gītā.* The sun-god is the origin of the *kṣatriyas*. If the king follows the instructions of the *Vedas* or other scriptures through the *brāhmaṇas,* or through a bona fide church, he is not only a king but a saintly person as well, a *rājarṣi*. The *kṣatriyas* should follow the orders of the *brāhmaṇas,* and the *vaiśyas* should follow the orders of the *kṣatriyas.* The *śūdras* should follow the instructions of the three superior orders.

Disciple: Concerning the beauty of God, Aquinas writes: "God is beautiful in Himself and not in relation to some limited terminus. . . . It is clear that the beauty of all things is derived from the divine beauty. . . . God wishes to multiply His own beauty as far as possible, that is to say, by the communication of His likeness. Indeed, all things are made in order to imitate divine beauty in some fashion."

Śrīla Prabhupāda: Yes, God is the reservoir of all knowledge, beauty, strength, fame, renunciation, and wealth. God is the reservoir of everything, and therefore whatever we see that is beautiful emanates from a very minute part of God's beauty.

yad yad vibhūtimat sattvaṁ śrīmad ūrjitam eva vā
tat tad evāvagaccha tvaṁ mama tejo-'ṁśa-sambhavam

"Know that all opulent, beautiful, and glorious creations spring from but a spark of My splendor" [*Bhagavad-gītā* 10.41].

Disciple: Concerning the relationship between theology and philosophy, Aquinas writes: "As sacred doctrine is based on the light of faith, so is philosophy founded on the natural light of reason. . . . If any point among the statements of the philosophers is found contrary to faith, this is not philosophy but rather an abuse of philosophy, resulting from a defect in reasoning."

Śrīla Prabhupāda: Yes, that is correct. Due to material, conditioned life, every man is defective. The philosophy of defective people cannot help society. Perfect philosophy comes from one who is in contact with the Supreme Personality of Godhead, and such philosophy is beneficial. Speculative philosophers base their beliefs on imagination.

Disciple: Aquinas concluded that divine revelation is absolutely necessary because very few men can arrive at the truth through the philosophical method. It is a path full of errors, and the journey takes a long time.

Śrīla Prabhupāda: Yes, that is a fact. We should directly contact the Supreme Person, Kṛṣṇa, who has complete knowledge. We should understand His instructions and try to follow them.

Disciple: Aquinas believed that the author of sacred scripture can be only God Himself, who can not only "adjust words to their meaning, which even man can do, but also adjust things in themselves." Also, scriptures are not restricted to one meaning.

Śrīla Prabhupāda: The meaning of scriptures is one, but the interpretations may be different. In the Bible it is stated that God created the universe, and that is a fact. One may conjecture that the universe was created out of some chunk, or whatever, but we should not interpret scripture in this way. We present the *Bhagavad-gītā* as it is, without interpretation or motive. We cannot change the words of God. Unfortunately, many interpreters of scripture have spoiled the God consciousness of society.

Disciple: In this, Aquinas seems to differ from the official Catholic doctrine, which admits only the Pope's interpretation. For him, the scriptures may contain many meanings according to our degree of realization.

Śrīla Prabhupāda: The meaning is one, but if we are not realized, we may interpret many meanings. It is stated in both the Bible and the *Bhagavad-gītā* that God created the universe. In the *Gītā* we find that Lord Kṛṣṇa states, *ahaṁ sarvasya prabhavo mattaḥ sarvaṁ pravartate:* "I am the source of all spiritual and material worlds. Everything emanates from Me" [*Bhagavad-gītā* 10.8]. If it is a fact that everything is an emanation of God's energy, why should we accept a second meaning or interpretation? What is the possible second meaning?

Disciple: Well, in the Bible it is stated that after creating the universe, God walked through paradise in the afternoon. Aquinas would consider this to have an interior, or metaphorical, meaning.

Śrīla Prabhupāda: If God can create, He can also walk, speak, touch, and see. If God is a person, why is a second meaning necessary? What could it possibly be?

Disciple: Impersonal speculation.

Śrīla Prabhupāda: If God is the creator of all things, He must be a person. Things appear to come from secondary causes, but actually everything is created by the supreme creator.

Disciple: Aquinas seems to have encouraged individual inter-

pretation. He writes: "It belongs to the dignity of divine scripture to contain many meanings in one text, so that it may be appropriate to the various understandings of men for each man to marvel at the fact that he can find the truth that he has conceived in his own mind expressed in divine scripture."
Śrīla Prabhupāda: No. If one's mind is perfect, he may give a meaning, but, according to our conviction, if one is perfect, why should he try to change the word of God? And if one is imperfect, what is the value of his change?
Disciple: Aquinas doesn't say "change."
Śrīla Prabhupāda: Interpretation means change. If man is imperfect, how can he change the words of God? If the words can be changed, they are not perfect. So there will be doubt whether the words are spoken by God or by an imperfect person.
Disciple: The many different Protestant faiths resulted from such individual interpretation. It's surprising to find this viewpoint in Aquinas.
Śrīla Prabhupāda: As soon as you interpret or change the scripture, the scripture loses its authority. Then another man will come and interpret things in his own way. Another will come and then another, and in this way the original purport of the scripture is lost.
Disciple: Aquinas believed that it is not possible to see God in this life. He writes: "God cannot be seen in His essence by one who is merely man, except he be separated from this mortal life. . . . The divine essence cannot be known through the nature of material things."
Śrīla Prabhupāda: What does he mean by divine essence? For us, God's divine essence is personal. When one cannot conceive of the Personality of Godhead, he sees the impersonal feature everywhere. When one advances further, he sees God as the Paramātmā within his heart. That is the result of yoga meditation. Finally, if one is truly advanced, he can see God face to face. When Kṛṣṇa came, people saw him face to face. Christians accept Christ as the son of God, and when he came, people saw him face to face. Does Aquinas think that

Christ is not the divine essence of God?

Disciple: For a Christian, Christ must be the divine essence.

Śrīla Prabhupāda: And didn't many people see him? Then how can Aquinas say that God cannot be seen?

Disciple: It's difficult to tell whether Aquinas is basically impersonalist or personalist.

Śrīla Prabhupāda: That means he is speculating.

Disciple: He writes about the personal feature in this way: "Because God's nature has all perfection and thus every kind of perfection should be attributed to Him, it is fitting to use the word 'person' to speak of God; yet when used of God it is not used exactly as it is of creatures but in a higher sense. . . . Certainly the dignity of divine nature surpasses every nature, and thus it is entirely suitable to speak of God as a 'person.'" Aquinas is no more specific than this.

Śrīla Prabhupāda: Christ is accepted as the son of God, and if the son can be seen, why can't the Father be seen? If Christ is the son of God, who is God? In the *Bhagavad-gītā,* Kṛṣṇa says, *ahaṁ sarvasya prabhavaḥ:* "Everything is emanating from Me." Christ says that he is the son of God, and this means that he emanates from God. Just as he has his personality, God also has His personality. Therefore we refer to Kṛṣṇa as the Supreme Personality of Godhead.

Disciple: Concerning God's names, Aquinas writes: "Yet since God is simple and subsisting, we attribute to Him simple and abstract names to signify His simplicity, and concrete names to signify His subsistence and perfection; although both these kinds of names fail to express His mode of being, because our intellect does not know Him in this life as He is."

Śrīla Prabhupāda: One of God's attributes is being. Similarly, one of His attributes is attraction. God attracts everything. The word *kṛṣṇa* means "all-attractive." What, then, is wrong with addressing God as Kṛṣṇa? Because Kṛṣṇa is the enjoyer of Rādhārāṇī, His name is Rādhikā-ramaṇa. Because He exists, He is called the Supreme Being. In one sense, God has no name, but in another sense He has millions of names according to His activities and attributes.

Disciple: Aquinas maintains that although the names apply to God to signify one reality, they are not synonymous because they signify that reality under diverse aspects.

Śrīla Prabhupāda: God's names are there because He has different features and activities.

Disciple: But Aquinas asserts that no name belongs to God in the same sense that it belongs to creatures.

Śrīla Prabhupāda: The names of creatures are also derived from God. For instance, God appeared as the boar incarnation, and therefore a devotee may be named Varāha dāsa, which means "servant of God in His boar incarnation." This name is not created; it refers to the activities of God.

Disciple: Aquinas believed that names of God that imply relation to creatures are predicated of God temporarily. He writes: "Though God is prior to the creature, still, because the signification of 'Lord' includes the idea of a servant and vice versa, these two relative terms, Lord and servant, are simultaneous by nature. Hence God was not 'Lord' until He had a creature subject to Himself. . . . Thus names which import relation to creatures are applied to God temporarily, and not from eternity, since God is outside the whole order of creation."

Śrīla Prabhupāda: God is always existing as the Lord, and His servants are existing everlastingly with Him. How can He be the Lord without a servant? How can it be that God has no servants?

Disciple: Well, the contention is that creatures were created at one point in time, and before that, God must have been by Himself.

Śrīla Prabhupāda: That is a material idea. It is the material world that is created, not the spiritual world. The spiritual world and God are existing everlastingly. The bodies of creatures in this material world are created, but God is always in the spiritual world with countless servants. According to our philosophy, there is no limit to the number of living entities. Those who do not like to serve are put into this material world. As far as our identity as servants is concerned, that is eternal, whether we are in the material world or the spiritual world. If we do not serve God in the spiritual world, we come down into the material world to serve the illusory energy of God. In any case, God is always the master, and the living entity is always the servant.

Disciple: Aquinas felt that the less determinate God's name, the more universal and absolute it is. He therefore believed that the most proper name for God is "He who is."

Śrīla Prabhupāda: Why? If God is active and has created the entire universe, what is wrong in addressing Him according to His activities and attributes?

Disciple: Aquinas claims that the very essence of God is the sheer fact of His being, the fact that He is.

Śrīla Prabhupāda: He is, certainly, but "He is" means that He is existing in His abode with His servants, playmates, hobbies, and paraphernalia. Everything is there. We must ask what is the meaning or nature of His being.

Disciple: It seems that Aquinas was basically an impersonalist.

Śrīla Prabhupāda: No. He could not determine whether God is personal or impersonal. His inclination was to serve God as a person, but he had no clear conception of His personality. Therefore he speculated.

Disciple: In the *Vedas,* is there an equivalent to "He who is"?

Śrīla Prabhupāda: *Oṁ tat sat* is impersonal. This *mantra,* however, can also be extended as *oṁ namo bhagavate vāsudevāya.* The word *vāsudeva* means "one who lives everywhere" and refers to Bhagavān, the Supreme Personality of Godhead. God is both personal and impersonal, but the impersonal feature is secondary. According to Bhagavān Śrī Kṛṣṇa in the *Bhagavad-gītā:*

> *brahmaṇo hi pratiṣṭhāham amṛtasyāvyayasya ca*
> *śāśvatasya ca dharmasya sukhasyaikāntikasya ca*

"And I am the basis of the impersonal Brahman, which is

immortal, imperishable, and eternal and is the constitutional position of ultimate happiness" [*Bhagavad-gītā* 14.27]. What is the purport to that?

Disciple [reading]: "The constitution of Brahman is immortality, imperishability, eternity, and happiness. Brahman is the beginning of transcendental realization. Paramātmā, the Supersoul, is the middle, the second stage in transcendental realization, and the Supreme Personality of Godhead is the ultimate realization of the Absolute Truth."

Śrīla Prabhupāda: That is divine essence.

Jean-Paul Sartre: Is the Supreme Being Nothingness?

Jean-Paul Sartre (1905–1980) was perhaps the most prominent exponent of existentialism in the twentieth century.

Disciple: Descartes and Leibnitz believed that before the creation the concept of man existed in essence in the mind of God, just as a machine exists in the mind of its manufacturer before it is constructed. Sartre takes exception to this. In *The Humanism of Existentialism,* he writes: "Atheistic existentialism, which I represent, is more coherent. It states that if God does not exist, there is at least one being in whom existence precedes essence, a being who exists before he can be defined by any concept, and that this being is man, or, as Heidegger says, human reality."
Śrīla Prabhupāda: But where does human reality come from? There are also other realities. Why is he stressing human reality?
Disciple: As for man's origin, Sartre would say that man is "thrown into the world."
Śrīla Prabhupāda: Thrown by whom? The word "throw" implies a thrower.
Disciple: Sartre isn't really interested in a thrower. "Existentialism isn't so atheistic that it wears itself out showing God doesn't exist," he writes. "Rather, it declares that even if God did exist, that would change nothing. There you've got our point of view. Not that we believe that God exists, but that we think that the problem of His existence is not the issue."
Śrīla Prabhupāda: But if you and others exist, why doesn't God exist? Why deny God and His existence? Let them all exist.
Disciple: Since Sartre sees man as having been thrown into the world and abandoned, for him, God is dead.
Śrīla Prabhupāda: Abandoned by God does not mean that God is dead. You have to admit that you are condemned to

the material world, but just because you are condemned, you should not think that God is also condemned. God is always in Vaikuṇṭha. He is not dead.

Disciple: Sartre believes that because we have been abandoned, we must rely on ourselves alone.

Śrīla Prabhupāda: But God has not abandoned us. God is not partial. He does not accept one person and abandon another. If you feel abandoned, it is because you have done something that has brought this condition about. If you rectify your position, you will be accepted again.

Disciple: But Sartre would deny God's existence, particularly that of a personal God. This is evident from his main book, *Being and Nothingness.*

Śrīla Prabhupāda: But his denial should be based on some logic or reason. Why mention the word "God" if God does not exist? God is there, but Sartre denies God's existence. This is inconsistent. If God does not exist, why even mention the word? His proposal is that he does not want God to exist.

Disciple: He wants to set the whole question aside in order to place emphasis on man, on human reality.

Śrīla Prabhupāda: If you believe in your existence, why not believe in the existence of another? There are 8,400,000 different species existing in multifarious forms. Why shouldn't God exist? According to the Vedic understanding, God is also a living being, but He is different in that He is the chief, supreme living being. According to the *Bhagavad-gītā, mattaḥ parataraṁ nānyat* [*Bhagavad-gītā* 7.7]. There is no living being superior to God. We all experience the fact that there are beings more intelligent than we. God is the ultimate intelligence. Why can't a person who exceeds all others in intelligence exist? There is no question of "if God exists." God *must* exist. In the *śāstras* He is described as the superlative personality, as the super-powerful, super-intelligent being. We can see in this world that everyone is not on an equal level, that there are varying degrees of perfection. This indicates that there is a superlative, and if we go on searching—either for wealth, intelligence, power, beauty, or whatever—

we will find that God possesses all qualities to the superlative degree, and that every other living entity possesses His qualities partially. How, then, can we rationally deny His existence?

Disciple: According to Sartre, the first principle of existentialism is that "man is nothing else but what he makes of himself." This can be true only if there is no God to conceive of human nature.

Śrīla Prabhupāda: If man is what he makes of himself, why doesn't man exist as a superman? If his capacities are completely independent of anyone else, why is he in his present situation?

Disciple: That is also Sartre's question. He therefore emphasizes man's responsibility. "But if existence really does precede essence," he writes, "man is responsible for what he is. Thus existentialism's first move is to make every man aware of what he is and to make the full responsibility of his existence rest on him."

Śrīla Prabhupāda: If man is responsible, who gave him this responsibility? What does he mean by responsibility? You feel responsible to someone when someone gives you duties to discharge. If there is no duty, or overseer, where is your responsibility?

Disciple: Sartre sees man as being overwhelmed by his very responsibility. He is in anguish and anxiety because he has the freedom to change himself and the world.

Śrīla Prabhupāda: This means that man is in an awkward position. He wants peace, but he does not know how to attain it. But this does not mean that peace is not possible. Peace is not possible for a man in ignorance.

Disciple: Anxiety arises from responsibility. Man thinks that he has to choose properly in order to enjoy something. If he chooses wrongly, he must suffer.

Śrīla Prabhupāda: Yes, responsibility is there, but why not take it to transfer yourself to a safe place where there is no anxiety? It may be that you do not know of a safe place, but if there is such a place, why not ask someone who knows? Why constantly remain disappointed and anxious? The safe place where there is no anxiety is called Vaikuṇṭha. The word Vaikuṇṭha means "no anxiety."

Disciple: Sartre believes that the task of existentialism is "to make every man aware of what he is and to make the full responsibility of his existence rest on him. . . . And when we say that a man is responsible for himself, we do not only mean that he is responsible for his own individuality, but that he is responsible for all men."

Śrīla Prabhupāda: Suppose I want to benefit you, and you are free. Your freedom means that you can accept or reject my good intentions. How can I be responsible for you if you don't obey? How can you be responsible for me? Sartre claims that you are responsible for others, but if others do not follow your instructions, how can you be considered responsible? This is all contradictory. Unless there is some standard, there must be contradiction. According to the Vedic version, God is the Supreme Person, and we should all be His obedient servants. God gives us some duty, and we are responsible to carry that duty out. Our real responsibility is to God. If we reject God, society becomes chaotic. Religion means avoiding chaos and meeting our responsibility to God by fulfilling our duty. Responsibility rests on us, and it is given by God. If we make spiritual progress by fulfilling our duty, we can finally live with God personally.

Disciple: Sartre claims that the existentialist does not actually want to deny God's existence. Rather, "the existentialist thinks it very distressing that God does not exist because all possibility of finding values in a heaven of ideas disappears along with Him. . . . If God didn't exist, everything would be possible. That is the very starting point of existentialism. Indeed, everything is permissible if God does not exist. . . ."

Śrīla Prabhupāda: This means that he does not know the meaning of God. As we have many times said, God is the Supreme Being, the Supreme Father who impregnates material nature with countless living entities. As soon as we accept material nature as the mother, we must accept some father.

Therefore there is a conception of God the Father in all human societies. It is the father's duty to maintain his children, and therefore God is maintaining all the living entities within the universe. There is no question of rationally denying this.

Disciple: Well, Sartre at least makes the attempt. He writes: "Since we have discarded God the Father, there has to be someone to invent values. You've got to take things as they are. Moreover, to say that we invent values means nothing else but this: Life has no meaning a priori. Before you become alive, life is nothing; it's up to you to give it a meaning, and value is nothing else but the meaning that you choose."

Śrīla Prabhupāda: Therefore everyone invents his own meaning? If this is the case, how will people ever live peacefully in society? Since everyone has his own idea of life, there can be no harmony. What kind of government would exist?

Disciple: At one point Sartre turned to Marxism.

Śrīla Prabhupāda: But in Communist countries, there are very strong governments. It is not possible for a people to avoid government or leadership.

Disciple: Regardless of the form of government, Sartre believes that man is basically free. In fact, Sartre maintains that man is *condemned* to be free, that this is a fate from which man cannot escape.

Śrīla Prabhupāda: If man is condemned, who has condemned him?

Disciple: Man is condemned by accident, thrown into the world.

Śrīla Prabhupāda: Is it simply by accident that one person is condemned and another blessed? Is it an accident that one man is in jail and another is not? What kind of philosophy is this? Such so-called philosophy simply misleads people. Nothing is accidental. We agree that the living entity is condemned to this material world, but when we speak of condemnation, we also speak of blessedness. So what is that blessedness?

Disciple: Sartre argues that man is condemned in the sense that he cannot escape this freedom. Since man is free,

he is responsible for his actions.
Śrīla Prabhupāda: If you are responsible, then your freedom is not accidental. How is it you are accidentally responsible? If there is responsibility, there must be someone you are responsible to. There must be someone who is condemning you or blessing you. These things cannot happen accidentally. His philosophy is contradictory.
Disciple: Man's nature is an indefinite state of freedom. Man has no definite nature. He is continually creating it.
Śrīla Prabhupāda: This means that he is eternal. But the living entity does not change accidentally. His changes take place under certain regulations, and he attains specific bodies according to his *karma,* not by accident.
Disciple: But we have no fixed nature in the sense that today I may be happy and tomorrow unhappy.
Śrīla Prabhupāda: That is true to some extent. When you are placed into the sea, you have no control. You move according to the waves. This means that there is a power that is controlling you. However, if you put yourself in better circumstances, you will be able to control. Because you have placed yourself under the control of material nature, you act according to the modes of material nature.

prakṛteḥ kriyamāṇāni guṇaiḥ karmāṇi sarvaśaḥ
ahaṅkāra-vimūḍhātmā kartāham iti manyate

"The spirit soul bewildered by the influence of false ego thinks himself the doer of activities that are in actuality carried out by the three modes of material nature" [*Bhagavad-gītā* 3.27]. Because you are conditioned, your freedom is checked. When you are thrown into the ocean of material existence, you essentially lose your freedom. Therefore it is your duty to get yourself liberated.
Disciple: Because we are one thing today and something else tomorrow, Sartre says that our essential nature is "no-thingness."
Śrīla Prabhupāda: You are nothing in the sense that you are

under the full control of a superior power, being carried away by the waves of *māyā*. In the ocean of *māyā,* you may say, "I am nothing," but actually you are something. Your something-ness will be very much exhibited to you when you are put on land. Out of despair, you conclude that your nature is that of nothingness. Sartre's philosophy is a philosophy of despair, and we say that it is unintelligent because despair is not the result of intelligence.

Disciple: Although the basis of our nature is nothingness, Sartre maintains that man chooses or creates his own nature.

Śrīla Prabhupāda: That is a fact. Therefore you should create your nature as something, not nothing. In order to do that, however, you have to take lessons from a higher personality. Before philosophizing, Sartre should have taken lessons from a knowledgeable person. That is the Vedic injunction:

tad-vijñānārthaṁ sa gurum evābhigacchet
samit-pāṇiḥ śrotriyaṁ brahma-niṣṭham

"In order to learn the transcendental science, one must humbly approach a spiritual master who is learned in the *Vedas* and firmly devoted to the Absolute Truth" [*Muṇḍaka Upaniṣad* 1.2.12].

Disciple: Sartre sees our nature as always in the making, as continually becoming.

Śrīla Prabhupāda: It is not in the making. It is changing. But man can make his nature in the sense that he can decide not to change. He can understand that changes are taking place despite the fact that he does not want them. Man can mold his nature by deciding to serve Kṛṣṇa, not by dismissing the whole matter and, out of confusion and disappointment, claiming to be nothing. The attempt to make life zero is due to a poor fund of knowledge.

Disciple: Sartre sees that we are constantly choosing or making our life, but that everything ends at death. That is, man is always in the process of becoming until death. At death, everything is finished.

Śrīla Prabhupāda: Death means changing into another body. The active principle on which the body stands does not die. Death is like changing apartments. A sane man can understand this.

Disciple: Although man has no determined nature other than nothingness, Sartre sees man as a being striving to be God. He writes: "To be man means to reach toward being God. Or if you prefer, man fundamentally is the desire to be God."

Śrīla Prabhupāda: On the one hand, he denies the existence of God, and on the other, he tries to be God. If there is no God, there is no question of desiring to be God. How can one desire to be something that does not exist?

Disciple: He is simply stating that man wants to be God. As far as God's existence is concerned, he prefers to set this question aside.

Śrīla Prabhupāda: But that is the main question of philosophy! God has created everything: your mind, intelligence, body, existence, and the circumstances surrounding you. How can you deny His existence? Or set it aside as not relevant? In the *Vedas,* it is stated that in the beginning God existed, and the Bible also states that in the beginning there was God. In this material universe, existence and annihilation are both temporary. According to the laws of material nature, the body is created on a certain day, it exists for some time, and then it is eventually finished. The entire cosmic manifestation has a beginning, middle, and end, But before this creation, who was there? If God were not there, how could the creation logically be possible?

Disciple: As far as we've seen, most philosophers are concerned with resolving this question.

Śrīla Prabhupāda: Not all philosophers are denying God's existence, but most are denying His personal existence. We can understand, however, that God is the origin of everything, and that this cosmic manifestation emanates from Him. God is there, nature is there, and we are also there, like one big family.

Disciple: Sartre would not admit the existence of an originator in whom things exist in their essence prior to creation. He would say that man simply exists, that he just appears.

Śrīla Prabhupāda: A person appears due to his father and mother. How can this be denied? Does he mean to say, "I suddenly just dropped from the sky"? Only a fool would say that he appeared without parents. From our experience we can understand that all species of life are manifest from some mother. Taken as a whole, we say that the mother is material nature. As soon as a mother is accepted, the father must also be accepted. It is most important to know where you came from. How can you put this question aside?

Disciple: Sartre believes that man's fundamental desire is the "desire to be." That is, man seeks existence rather than mere nothingness.

Śrīla Prabhupāda: That is so. Because man is eternal, he has the desire to exist eternally. Unfortunately, he puts himself under certain conditions that are not eternal. That is, he tries to maintain a position that will not endure eternally. Through Kṛṣṇa consciousness, we attain and retain our eternal position.

Disciple: Sartre feels that man wants solidity. He is not satisfied with being a mere being-for-itself. He also desires to be being-*in*-itself.

Śrīla Prabhupāda: Nothing in the material world exists eternally. A tree may exist for ten thousand years, but eventually it will perish. What Sartre is seeking is actual spiritual life. In the *Bhagavad-gītā,* Kṛṣṇa speaks of another nature, a nature that is permanent, *sanātana.*

paras tasmāt tu bhāvo 'nyo 'vyakto 'vyaktāt sanātanaḥ
yaḥ sa sarveṣu bhūteṣu naśyatsu na vinaśyati

"Yet there is another unmanifest nature, which is eternal and is transcendental to this manifested and unmanifested matter. It is supreme and is never annihilated. When all in this world is annihilated, that part remains as it is" [*Bhagavad-gītā* 8.20]. After the annihilation of this material

universe, that eternal nature will abide.
Disciple: This desire to be being-in-itself is the desire to be God, which Sartre maintains is man's fundamental desire.
Śrīla Prabhupāda: This is more or less Māyāvādī philosophy. The Māyāvādīs believe that when they attain complete knowledge, they become God. Because man is part and parcel of God, he wants to be united with God. It is like a man who has been away from home for a long time. Naturally he wants to go home again.
Disciple: Sartre believes that this desire to be God is bound to fail.
Śrīla Prabhupāda: Certainly, it must fail. If man is God, how has he become something else? His very desire to be God means that he is not God at the present moment. A man cannot become God, but he can become god*ly*. Existing in darkness, we desire light. We may come into the sunshine, but this does not mean that we become the sun. When we come to the platform of perfect knowledge, we become godly, but we do not become God. If we were God, there would be no question of our becoming something other than God. There would be no question of being ignorant. Another name for Kṛṣṇa is Acyuta, which means, "He who never falls down." This means that He never becomes not-God. He is God always. You cannot become God through some mystic practice. This desire to become God is useless because it is doomed to frustration.
Disciple: Therefore Sartre calls man a "useless passion."
Śrīla Prabhupāda: A man is not useless if he attempts to be Kṛṣṇa conscious. The attempt to be Kṛṣṇa conscious and the attempt to be Kṛṣṇa are totally different. One is godly, the other demoniac.
Disciple: Sartre then reasons that because it is impossible to become God, everything else is useless.
Śrīla Prabhupāda: That is foolishness. You are not God, but God's servant. You have chosen to attempt to become God, but you have found this to be impossible. Therefore you should give up this notion and decide to become a good ser-

vant of God, instead of a servant of *māyā,* illusion. That is the proper decision.

Disciple: Sartre concludes that since things have no reason to exist, life has no essential purpose.

Śrīla Prabhupāda: Nothing can exist without a purpose, which is given by the supreme being, the cause of all causes. The defect in such philosophers is that they do not have sufficient brain substance to go further than what they superficially see. They are not capable of understanding the cause of all causes. Many modern scientists also maintain that nature, *prakṛti,* is the sole cause of existence, but we do not ascribe to such a theory. We understand that God is behind nature, and that nature is not acting independently. Nature is phenomena, but behind nature is numina, God, Kṛṣṇa.

In the *Bhagavad-gītā,* philosophy like Sartre's is called demoniac. Demons do not believe in a superior cause. They consider that everything is accidental. They say that a man and a woman unite accidentally, and that their child is the result of sex and nothing more. Therefore they claim that there is no purpose to existence.

asatyam apratiṣṭhaṁ te jagad āhur anīśvaram
aparaspara-sambhūtaṁ kim anyat kāma-haitukam

"They say that this world is unreal, with no foundation, no God in control. They say it is produced of sex desire and has no cause other than lust" [*Bhagavad-gītā* 16.8]. This type of philosophy is called demoniac because it is of the nature of darkness, ignorance.

Disciple: For Sartre, being-for-itself refers to human consciousness, which is subjective, individual, incomplete, and indeterminate. It is nothingness in the sense that it has no density or mass.

Śrīla Prabhupāda: Because he is so materialistic, his senses cannot perceive anything that is not concrete. According to Vedic philosophy, the senses and their objects are created simultaneously. Unless there is an aroma, the sense of smell has no value. Unless there is beauty, the eyes have no value. Unless there is music, the ears have no value. Unless there is something soft, the sense of touch has no value. There is no question of nothingness. There must be interaction.

Disciple: Since man's essential nature is an undetermined nothingness, Sartre believes that man is free to choose to be either a coward or a hero. Our situation is in our own hands.

Śrīla Prabhupāda: If you are tossed into the world by some superior power, what can you do? How can you become a hero? If you try to become a hero, you will be kicked all the more because you are placed here by a superior power. If a culprit under police custody attempts to become a hero, he will be beaten and punished. Actually, you are neither a coward nor a hero. You are an instrument. You are completely under the control of a superior power.

Disciple: Well, if someone is attacking you, you have the power to choose to be a hero and defend yourself, or to run.

Śrīla Prabhupāda: It is not heroic to defend oneself. That is natural. If that is the case, even a dog can be a hero when he is attacked. Even an ant can be a hero. Heroism and cowardice are simply mental concoctions. After all, you are under the control of a power that can do what He likes with you. Therefore there is no question of your becoming a hero or a coward.

Disciple: Suppose someone is in danger, and you rescue him. Isn't that being heroic?

Śrīla Prabhupāda: All you rescue is the exterior dress. Saving that dress is not heroism. It is not even protection. One can be a real hero only when he is fully empowered or fully protected. Such a person can only be a devotee, because only Kṛṣṇa can fully protect or empower.

Disciple: Being free, man is subject to what Sartre calls "bad faith," a kind of self-deception. Through bad faith, man loses his freedom and responsibility.

Śrīla Prabhupāda: You certainly have limited freedom to choose, but if you choose improperly, you have to suffer. Responsibility and freedom go hand in hand. At the same time, there must be discrimination. Without it, our freedom is blind. We cannot understand right from wrong.

Disciple: A man in bad faith drifts along from day to day without being involved, avoiding responsible decisions.

Śrīla Prabhupāda: This means that he has decided to drift. His drifting is a decision.

Disciple: Sartre believes that bad faith must be replaced by a solid choosing, and by faith in that choice.

Śrīla Prabhupāda: But if he makes the wrong decision, what is the value of his action? Moths fly very valiantly and courageously into the fire. Is that a very good decision?

Disciple: Due to bad faith, people treat others as objects instead of persons. Sartre advocates rectifying this situation.

Śrīla Prabhupāda: He speaks of bad faith, but what about good faith?

Disciple: If bad faith is the avoidance of decisions, good faith would mean making decisions courageously and following them out, regardless of what these decisions are.

Śrīla Prabhupāda: But what if your decision is wrong?

Disciple: For Sartre, it is not a question of right or wrong.

Śrīla Prabhupāda: Then whatever decision I make is final and absolute? This means that the moth's decision to enter the fire is a proper decision. This is the philosophy of insects. If man can do as he pleases, where is his responsibility?

Disciple: Sartre believes that the fate of the world depends on man's decisions. Obviously, if man decides properly, the world would be a better place.

Śrīla Prabhupāda: Therefore we are trying to introduce this Kṛṣṇa consciousness in order to make the world into Vaikuṇṭha, into a place where there is no anxiety. But this is not a blind decision. It is the decision of a higher authority; therefore it is perfect.

Disciple: Many people call Sartre's philosophy pessimistic because he maintains that man is a "useless passion" vainly striving in a universe without a purpose.

Śrīla Prabhupāda: Sartre may be a useless passion, but we are not. No sane man is useless. A sane man will follow a superior authority. That is Vedic civilization. If one approaches a bona fide spiritual master, he will not be bewildered. Sartre believes that the universe is without a purpose because he is blind. He has no power to see that there is a plan. Therefore, as I have already mentioned, the *Bhagavad-gītā* calls his philosophy demoniac. Everything in the universe functions according to some plan. The sun and moon rise, and the seasons change according to plan.

Disciple: For Sartre, man stands alone in the world, yet he is not alone if he is a being-for-others. Man needs others for his own self-realization.

Śrīla Prabhupāda: This means that man requires a guru.

Disciple: Sartre does not speak of a guru but of interaction with others for self-understanding.

Śrīla Prabhupāda: If this is required, why not interact with the best man? If we require others to understand ourselves, why should we not seek the best man for our own understanding? We should receive help from the man who knows. If you take the advice of one who can give you the right direction, your end will be glorious. That is the Vedic injunction. *Tad-vijñānārthaṁ sa gurum evābhigacchet* [*Muṇḍaka Upaniṣad* 1.2.12].

Disciple: Sartre feels that in the presence of others, man is ashamed.

Śrīla Prabhupāda: Man is ashamed if he is not guided by a superior. If you are guided by a superior, you will be glorious, not ashamed. Your superior is that person who can lead you to the glory of Kṛṣṇa consciousness.

Give God the Nobel Prize

On an early-morning walk, Śrīla Prabhupāda points out to his disciples how insignificant are man's scientific achievements compared to God's limitlessly complex creation. (June 1974, Geneva)

Śrīla Prabhupāda: Just look at this fig. In this one fig, you find thousands of seeds—and each tiny seed can produce another tree as big as the original fig tree. Inside each little seed is a whole new fig tree.

Now, where is that chemist who can do such a thing: first, make a tree, and then, make the tree bear fruit, and next, make the fruit produce seeds—and finally, make the seeds produce still more trees? Just tell me. Where is that chemist?

Disciple: They talk very proudly, Śrīla Prabhupāda, but none of these chemists and such can do any of these things.

Śrīla Prabhupāda: Once a big chemist came to me and admitted, "Our chemical advancement, our scientific advancement, is like a man who has learned to bark. So many natural dogs are already barking, but no one pays any attention. But if a man artificially learns the art of barking, oh, so many people will go to see—and even purchase tickets for ten dollars, twenty dollars. Just to see an artificial dog. Our scientific advancement is like this."

If a man makes an artificial imitation of nature, say by barking, people go to see and even pay money. When it comes to the natural barking, no one cares. And when these big so-called scientific rascals claim they can manufacture life, people give all sorts of praise and awards. As for God's perfect, natural process—millions and millions of beings born at each moment—no one cares. People don't give God's process very much credit.

The fool who concocts some imaginary scheme for creating living beings from dead material chemicals—he is given all credit, you see: the Nobel Prize. "Oh, here is a creative genius." And nature is injecting millions and millions of souls into material bodies at every moment—by the arrangement of God—and no one cares. This is rascaldom.

Even if we suppose you *could* manufacture a man or animal in your laboratory, what would be your credit? After all, a single man or animal might be created by you, but millions and millions are created by the Lord. So we want to give credit to Kṛṣṇa, who is really creating all these living beings we see every day.

Disciple: Prabhupāda, you remember Aldous Huxley, who in *Brave New World* predicted a process of genetically screening babies, of breeding men for certain traits? The idea would be to take one strain of traits and breed a class of working men, take another strain of traits and breed a class of administrators, and take still another strain of traits and breed a class of cultured advisors and scholars.

Śrīla Prabhupāda: Once again, that is already present in God's natural arrangement. *Guṇa-karma-vibhāgaśaḥ:* according to one's qualities and activities in his past life, in his present life he gets a fitting body. If one has cultivated the qualities and activities of ignorance, he gets an ignorant body and must live by manual labor. If one has cultivated the qualities and activities of striving passion, he gets a passionate body and must live by taking charge of others—administration.

If one has cultivated the qualities and activities of enlightenment, he gets an enlightened body and must live by enlightening and advising others.

So you see, God has already made such a perfect arrangement. Every soul receives the body he desires and deserves, and the social order receives citizens with required traits. Not that you have to "breed" these traits. By His natural arrangement, the Lord equips particular souls with particular kinds of bodies. Why even try imitating what God and nature already do perfectly?

I told that scientist who visited me, "You scientists—you are simply wasting time." Childish. They are just imitating the dog's barking. The scientist pays no attention, gives no credit to the real dog doing the real barking. Actually, that is today's situation. When the natural dog barks, that is not science. When the artificial, imitation dog barks, that is science. Isn't it so? To whatever degree the scientist succeeds in artificially imitating what the Lord's natural arrangement is already doing—that is science.

Disciple: When you heard, Prabhupāda, about the scientists claiming they can now produce babies in a test tube, you said, "But that is already being done in the mother's womb. The womb is the perfect test tube."

Śrīla Prabhupāda: Yes. Nature is already doing everything with utter perfection. But some puffed-up scientist will make a shabby imitation—using the ingredients nature supplies—and get the Nobel Prize.

And what to speak of actually creating a baby—let us see the scientists produce even one blade of grass in their proud laboratories.

Disciple: They should give the Lord and Mother Nature the Nobel Prize.

Śrīla Prabhupāda: Yes, yes.

Disciple: Really, I think they should give you the Nobel Prize. You've taken so many foolish atheists and created devotees of God.

Śrīla Prabhupāda: Oh, I—I am a "natural dog," so they'll not give me any prize. [*Laughs.*] They will award the prize to the artificial dogs.

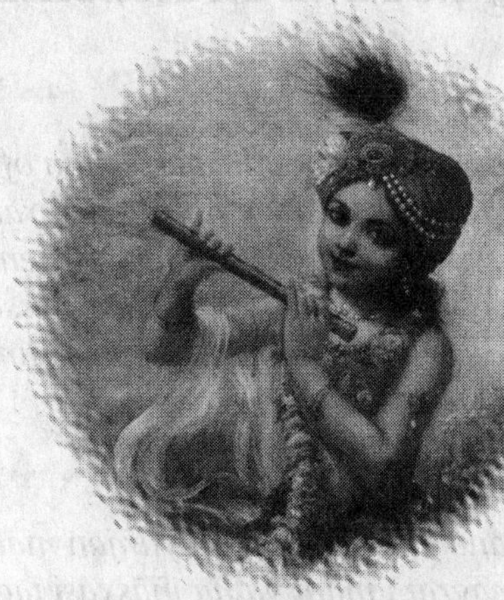

7.

Love of God, The Ultimate Goal

The Yoga of Pure Attachment

Here Śrīla Prabhupāda describes the perfection of yoga: "Why does the river flow to the sea? It is simply natural; there is no artificial reason why it flows there. Similarly, when our love for Kṛṣṇa will glide down like that, without any personal motive, we will have achieved perfection in yoga." (June 1972, San Diego, California)

śrī-bhagavān uvāca
mayy āsakta-manāḥ pārtha yogaṁ yuñjan mad-āśrayaḥ
asaṁśayaṁ samagraṁ māṁ yathā jñāsyasi tac chṛṇu

"The Supreme Personality of Godhead said, 'Now hear, O son of Pṛthā, how by practicing yoga in full consciousness of Me, with your mind attached to Me, you can know Me in full, free from doubt'" [*Bhagavad-gītā* 7.1].

The yoga system Kṛṣṇa mentions here is very simple and sublime. You have to simply engage your mind in thinking only of Kṛṣṇa, of the form of Kṛṣṇa. And how should you think of Him? With attachment (*āsakti*). If you love somebody, you always want to see him; your attachment is so strong that if you don't see him you become restless. Different people have different attachments, but attachment is always there.

Śrīla Rūpa Gosvāmī has explained very simply how we should be attached to God. He says, "My dear Lord, as a young man awakens his attachment immediately upon seeing a young girl, or as a young girl becomes attracted as soon as she sees a young boy, let me become attached to You." This kind of attachment is natural. Nobody has to go to the university to learn it.

Simply by seeing a young girl, a young boy thinks, "Oh, here is a nice, beautiful girl." And a young girl thinks, "Oh, here is a nice, beautiful boy." Similarly, we should think, "Oh, here is Kṛṣṇa, here are Kṛṣṇa's devotees, here are topics about Kṛṣṇa, here is Kṛṣṇa's temple."

Another example is that our attachment should flow toward Kṛṣṇa like the current of a river. A river automatically flows down to the sea. Just as the river is flowing toward the sea spontaneously, without any artificial attempt, our love should spontaneously flow toward Kṛṣṇa, or God. That is the perfection of yoga.

Yoga means "connection." In the beginning we may revive our connection with Kṛṣṇa artificially, but when that connection comes spontaneously, without any check, just like the river water going down incessantly to the sea, then we will be perfect in yoga. Nobody can check the flowing river. Why does the river flow to the sea? It is simply natural; there is no artificial reason why it flows there. Similarly, when our love for Kṛṣṇa will glide down like that, without any personal motive, we will have achieved perfection in yoga.

Spontaneous love for God does not depend on any external cause. Its only cause is the love itself. Therefore it is called *ahaitukī*. *Ahaitukī* means "without any cause or motive." Generally people go to a temple or church with a personal motive to fulfill. For example, the Christians go to church and pray, "God, give us our daily bread." The motive is the desire for bread. But when you go to church without any motive except to glorify God, that is real love. Of course, it is also nice to think, "God will give me bread; therefore let me go to church." But this motivated faith may be lost. If we approach God for some material benefit, our faith in Him may break at any time. So that is not the platform of real love of God. Real love is without personal motivation.

And this love is also *apratihatā*, "unable to be checked." Real love for God cannot be checked by any material condition. Nobody should say, "Because I am a poor man I have to work very hard, so I cannot love God now." People often talk like that: "I shall wait. When I get millions of dollars in my bank account I shall take to Kṛṣṇa consciousness. Now let me earn money." This is not *bhakti*. This is not attachment to Kṛṣṇa.

Here Kṛṣṇa says we should practice yoga under His protection (*mad-āśrayaḥ*). This means we must take shelter of Kṛṣṇa or His representative and try to practice that yoga by which we will attain spontaneous love for Kṛṣṇa. So, to awaken that attachment there are some regulative principles we must follow. For instance, we say, "No illicit sex." The Vedic system teaches that one who wants to have sex must get married and live according to religious principles. Then the husband and the wife can satisfy their desire for sex by begetting good children. There is no prohibition against sex; it is allowed. But not *illicit* sex. Engaging in illicit sex means you increase your attachment for sex, not Kṛṣṇa. Therefore it is forbidden.

Also, no meat-eating. Meat- or fish- or egg-eating—any nonvegetarian diet—is simply an attachment of the tongue. Nobody dies from not eating meat. That's a fact. When we were babies we depended on milk, either our mother's breast-milk or cow's milk. Therefore the cow is also our mother. Just as we drink breast-milk from our mother, we drink milk from mother cow. You must not kill your mother; that is a great sin. Therefore meat-eating is prohibited. But people have become so sinful that they do not consider, "When I was young this cow supplied her blood in the form of milk to feed me, to keep me alive. But now that I am grown up, I am so ungrateful that I am going to kill her and eat her flesh." This is the advancement of modern education: that people have learned how to kill their mother.

In every religion, killing is prohibited or very much restricted. In the Christian religion you have the commandment "Thou shalt not kill." But nearly everyone is violating this commandment. Then where is your claim to being a Christian? If you violate the injunction given by Lord Jesus Christ, how can you claim to be a Christian? That is our question. And even if one is not a Christian, killing is most sinful and should be avoided as far as possible.

Your first business in life is to increase your spontaneous attachment for God. That is the primary business of human life, because only in the human form of life can you do that. And as soon as you increase your attachment for Kṛṣṇa, your life is successful. "Successful" means that you won't have to accept any more material bodies. You will get a spiritual body and go to Kṛṣṇa—back home, back to Godhead. Therefore, if you increase your attachment for Kṛṣṇa, the benefit is that you make a solution to all the problems of your life.

To increase your attachment for Kṛṣṇa, in the beginning you have to follow some regulative principles, some restrictions. For instance, a doctor will prescribe a treatment: "Don't eat this. Don't do this." And he will say, "Do this." Similarly, in Kṛṣṇa consciousness there are so many do's and don't's. We have to accept the do's and avoid the don't's (*ānukūlyasya saṅkalpaḥ prātikūlyasya varjanam*). This is how to cultivate Kṛṣṇa consciousness favorably. We have to accept only those things favorable for awakening our attachment for Kṛṣṇa, and reject everything else.

So, if illicit sex is unfavorable for your advancement in Kṛṣṇa consciousness, you must reject it. You cannot argue. That will not help you. Similarly, you must reject intoxication, meat-eating, and gambling. Illicit sex, meat-eating, intoxication, and gambling—these are the four pillars of sinful life. The roof of sinful life is held up by these four pillars. In the beginning of Kṛṣṇa consciousness, when you are actually going to take Kṛṣṇa consciousness seriously, you must give up these four pillars of sinful life.

Today some souls will be initiated. This means that they are going to take up Kṛṣṇa consciousness very seriously. So, the first business of one who is serious to take up Kṛṣṇa consciousness is to break these four pillars of sinful life. Then there will be no chance of sin. As Kṛṣṇa says in the *Bhagavad-gītā* [7.28],

yeṣāṁ tv anta-gataṁ pāpaṁ janānāṁ puṇya-karmaṇām
te dvandva-moha-nirmuktā bhajante māṁ dṛḍha-vratāḥ

"One who has given up sinful activity and is simply engaging in pious activity—such a person is unbewildered and attains firm faith in Kṛṣṇa consciousness."

What are pious activities? first is *yajña,* performing some sacrifice. For example, today we are holding a fire sacrifice. Then another pious activity is giving charity for spreading Kṛṣṇa's propaganda. The Kṛṣṇa consciousness movement is making propaganda, so we require money. Money is Kṛṣṇa's energy. Everyone is holding Kṛṣṇa's money, and the sooner they spare some of that money for the sake of Kṛṣṇa, the better off they'll be. Suppose I am holding your money illegally. If I give it back to you, I become released from my criminal activities. Or suppose I have stolen something from your pocket and then I feel the pain of my conscience: "Oh, this stealing is not good." So, as soon as I return it to you, the thing is settled. But if I hold on to it, I am a criminal and will be punished. Similarly, all those persons who are holding Kṛṣṇa's money, not returning it to Kṛṣṇa, are criminals. And they will be punished.

How will they be punished? That we have seen. Recently there was a war between Pakistan and India. So, according to one's capacity, everyone in India had to contribute money to the war effort. All the rich men had to contribute fifty lakhs of rupees [about half a million dollars]. Many millions of rupees were collected and used to produce gunpowder—*Svāhā!**

So, if you don't execute *this svāhā,* you will have to execute *that svāhā.* The Vietnam War is going on—*Svāhā!* So many young men—*Svāhā!* So much money—*Svāhā!* Therefore, better learn how to make a *svāhā* for Kṛṣṇa. Otherwise you will have to make a *svāhā* for *māyā* [illusion].

So, one must perform sacrifice and give in charity for Kṛṣṇa. Then there is *tapasya. Tapasya* means voluntarily accepting all kinds of restrictive principles. Now we are addicted to all kinds of nonsense, but unless you stop all

---

**Svāhā* is a Sanskrit word spoken by the chief priest in a Vedic sacrifice as he pours clarified butter into the sacred fire, causing the fire to blaze up.

nonsensical activities, you cannot understand Kṛṣṇa consciousness. If you want to be serious, you must give them up.

In this way we have to increase our attachment for Kṛṣṇa. And if we increase our attachment for Kṛṣṇa, we will reach the perfection of yoga. Kṛṣṇa consciousness is the topmost yoga system. As Kṛṣṇa states in the *Bhagavad-gītā* [6.47], *yoginām api sarveṣāṁ mad-gatenāntarātmanā . . . sa me yuktatamo mataḥ:* "Of all yogis, one who is always thinking of Me is the best." You can always think of someone if you're attached to him. Otherwise, you cannot. It's not possible. If you love somebody, you will always see his picture, his form, in your mind. Always. As it is said in the Vedic literature, *premāñjana-cchurita-bhakti-vilocanena santaḥ sadaiva hṛdayeṣu vilokayanti.* We have to purify our eyes so we can see God within, and that purification is possible when we apply the ointment of love of God to our eyes daily. A doctor may prescribe that we apply some ointment to improve our eyesight. Similarly, you will see God when your vision is clarified by *premāñjana,* the ointment of love of God.

So, you must practice how to love Kṛṣṇa. First you have to rise early in the morning. You don't like to, but you think, "I will rise early to satisfy Kṛṣṇa." This is the beginning. Then, "I have to chant sixteen rounds of the Hare Kṛṣṇa *mantra* on my beads." You may be lazy, you may not want to do it, but if you want to love Kṛṣṇa you must do it. You must do it. In the beginning you have to learn how to love Kṛṣṇa, but when you actually come to the state of love of God there is no question of "have to." You will spontaneously follow the regulative principles, because love is there.

Learning to love Kṛṣṇa is something like developing love in our ordinary affairs. If I love a girl, I will give her a flower or other present. This is one of the six exchanges of love: you have to give a gift to your beloved. You also have to accept gifts from him (*dadāti pratigṛhṇāti*). Then *guhyam ākhyāti pṛcchati:* opening one's mind to the beloved. *Guhyam* means "very confidential things," and *ākhyāti* means "disclosing." You must disclose your innermost thoughts to your beloved, and he'll disclose his innermost thoughts to you. Then *bhuṅkte bhojayate caiva*—giving the lover something to eat and accepting food from him. These are the six ways of increasing love. If you act in these ways with Kṛṣṇa, you will develop love for Him.

Now we are taking so many things from Kṛṣṇa. Kṛṣṇa is giving us everything; all our necessities are being supplied by Him (*eko bahūnāṁ yo vidadhāti kāmān*). It is not possible to manufacture fruits, flowers, and grains in a factory. Kṛṣṇa is giving them to us. So, we are living at the cost of Kṛṣṇa, and if after cooking the grains we do not offer them to Kṛṣṇa, is that very gentlemanly?

In the Kṛṣṇa consciousness movement we cook food and then offer it to Kṛṣṇa. What is wrong with this? The rascals say, "These Kṛṣṇa conscious people are heathens because they offer food to a stone." Just see! These rascals are less intelligent. They do not know that God eats. As Kṛṣṇa says in the *Bhagavad-gītā* [9.26],

> *patraṁ puṣpaṁ phalaṁ toyaṁ yo me bhaktyā prayacchati*
> *tad ahaṁ bhakty-upahṛtam aśnāmi prayatātmanaḥ*

"When My devotee offers Me something within the categories of vegetables, grains, fruits, and water or milk, I eat it, because he has brought it with devotion and love." The devotee thinks, "Kṛṣṇa, You have given us so many nice foodstuffs, and I have cooked them. You please partake of the preparations first." This is love.

Suppose your father has given you many things, and you feel obliged to him. So when you cook something you will give it to him first, saying, "My dear father, I have cooked this. It is very nice, so please you eat it first." He will answer, "Oh, it is very nice? All right, give some to me." He will be so pleased with you. Actually, what you cook is already your father's property, so you cannot really give anything to him. Similarly, you don't actually have anything to offer to Kṛṣṇa. But if you become a little intelligent, you will offer Him back what already belongs to Him and in this way develop your love for Him. If you remain a rascal and steal God's property, your human life is spoiled, but if you become a little intelligent and offer everything back to Him, your life is successful.

God is giving us our daily bread, so why not offer it to Him first? That is intelligence. And rascaldom is to think, "God is giving me bread, so I shall eat it. That's all. I am meant only for eating." And why not for offering? We should feel gratitude toward God: "God has given me this bread, so let me offer it to Him first. Then I may eat." What is wrong with this idea? What is the loss? But the lowest of mankind do not even know that because God has given them something to eat, they should first offer it to Him before eating. And when you offer something to Kṛṣṇa, to God, He will eat it but then leave everything for you as *prasādam.* This is God's power.

So, *bhakti-yoga,* or Kṛṣṇa consciousness, is the process that will increase your attachment for Kṛṣṇa. We do not say, "Christians are bad, Hindus are good." No, we don't say that. We simply say, "Now in this human form of life, learn how to love God. For so long you have loved dog, now try to love God." That is our propaganda. We don't criticize anyone; we simply want to see whether he has developed his love for God. That's all. You can do it as a Christian, as a Hindu, or as a Muslim. We don't care. But we want to see whether you're actually a lover of God. If you are not, then we tell you, "Please try to love God in this way." What way is that? By *śravaṇaṁ kīrtanaṁ viṣṇoḥ*—simply hearing about Kṛṣṇa and chanting about Kṛṣṇa. Is that very difficult? If you have not yet learned how to love God, take up this process. If you simply hear about Kṛṣṇa in this temple, without doing anything else, your life will become perfect.

Thank you very much.

Bhakti—The Art of Eternal Love

In this lecture Śrīla Prabhupāda explains how we can awaken our dormant love for the supreme lovable object. (January 1973, Mumbai, India)

"The basic principle of the living condition is that we have a general propensity to love someone. No one can live without loving someone else. This propensity is present in every living being. Even an animal like a tiger has this loving propensity at least in a dormant stage, and it is certainly present in the human beings. The missing point, however, is where to repose our love so that everyone can become happy" [*The Nectar of Devotion,* Preface].

People become frustrated looking for the perfect object of love. We may love our brother and sister, our mother and father, our wife or husband, our friends, our community, our nation, the international community, or even all human beings, yet still our love will remain imperfect. That is because it is not all-inclusive. For example, every country considers the human beings residing there to be nationals, but not the animals. But "national" means anyone who takes birth in that country. In Sanskrit the word is *prajā,* "those who take birth." So it is the duty of the leader of a country to protect all *prajā* residing there. Not that only human beings should be protected, while the animals—the cows, pigs, chickens, and so on—are slaughtered. They are also *prajā.*

When one becomes Kṛṣṇa conscious, however, he loves every living being because of its connection with Kṛṣṇa. As Kṛṣṇa says, *sarva-yoniṣu kaunteya mūrtayaḥ sambhavanti yāḥ:* "Material nature is the mother of all forms of life, and I am the seed-giving father" [*Bhagavad-gītā* 14.4]. Real equality and brotherhood come when we see all living entities as equal, as children of the Lord. A person with such vision is called a *paṇḍita*, or wise man. A *paṇḍita* does not say, "Only my father and brother are good, and all others are bad." That is sectarianism. At present all the leaders are fools and rascals because they are simply sectarian, thinking, "I am good, my brother is good, my father is good, my countrymen are good, and all others are bad." That is the sum and substance of nationalism.

A devotee of Kṛṣṇa does not see like that. He does not like to kill even an ant. There was once a hunter named Mṛgāri who used to half-kill animals. After meeting the great sage Nārada, he became a devotee of Kṛṣṇa and was not prepared to kill even an ant. There is no partiality in a Vaiṣṇava [devotee of Kṛṣṇa]. He is everyone's friend, as Kṛṣṇa is everyone's friend. Just as Kṛṣṇa descends to reclaim all fallen souls back home, back to Godhead, similarly His representative, the devotee, also approaches everyone and tries to get them back home to Godhead. That includes even the animals. Once when Caitanya Mahāprabhu's party was going to Jagannātha Purī, a dog followed, and by his association with devotees the dog was also delivered.

We have a propensity to love, but we do not know how to make our love perfect. That perfection is possible when we love Kṛṣṇa. Now, in my old age, I am wandering all over the world teaching that everyone can become happy by practicing Kṛṣṇa consciousness. It is not that I love only my countrymen, only Hindus or Bengalis. I love everyone, even the animals. But because human beings can understand the Kṛṣṇa consciousness philosophy, I hold meetings for them. Yet whenever I get a chance, I give protection to the animals also. I give them *prasādam* [food offered to Kṛṣṇa]. I do not prohibit even an animal from coming to hear. They also hear sometimes. Everyone can hear.

Still, Kṛṣṇa consciousness is primarily for human beings. When properly trained in Kṛṣṇa consciousness, a human being can understand that Kṛṣṇa is present everywhere. An animal has no realization who Kṛṣṇa is, but a human being, after associating with devotees, can understand: "I know that the taste of the water I am drinking is Kṛṣṇa and that the light of the sun and moon are also Kṛṣṇa, because He states this in the *Bhagavad-gītā* [7.8]: *raso 'ham apsu kaunteya prabhāsmi śaśi-sūryayoḥ.*" In this way the person immediately remembers Kṛṣṇa, and that means he is also associating with Kṛṣṇa. When you hear about Kṛṣṇa, you are associating with Kṛṣṇa. When you chant about Kṛṣṇa, you are associating with Kṛṣṇa. When you remember Kṛṣṇa, you are associating with Kṛṣṇa.

The perfection of love of Kṛṣṇa is already there within everyone. As Lord Caitanya says,

nitya-siddha kṛṣṇa-prema 'sādhya' kabhu naya
śravaṇādi-śuddha-citte karaye udaya

"Pure love for Kṛṣṇa is eternally established in the hearts of all living entities. It is not something to be gained from another source. When one purifies his heart by hearing and chanting about Kṛṣṇa, that pure love naturally awakens" [*Caitanya-caritāmṛta, Madhya-līlā* 22.107].

A lump of gold is gold, though it may be covered with dirt. It simply has to be cleansed; then it becomes pure gold. Similarly, everyone is Kṛṣṇa conscious, but on account of association with matter people think they are something different from Kṛṣṇa. Because everyone is part and parcel of Kṛṣṇa, everyone has His qualities in minute degree, just as a speck of gold has the qualities of the vast mass of gold in the gold mine, or as a drop of sea water contains the same ingredients as the great ocean. The difference between Kṛṣṇa and us is that He is the great, unlimited spiritual being and we are infinitesimal particles of spirit.

On account of our association with *māyā,* the material energy, we have forgotten Kṛṣṇa. That forgetfulness is manifested by our desire to enjoy this material world. Everyone is trying to enjoy this world to his best capacity. Only the Kṛṣṇa conscious persons are not trying to enjoy this world but are trying to dovetail it in the service of Kṛṣṇa. That is the difference. For example, we eat *prasādam,* food offered to Kṛṣṇa. Everyone is eating, and we are also eating—but we do not eat directly after cooking. Whatever we prepare, we first offer to Kṛṣṇa. We cannot manufacture rice, beans, wheat, fruit, or milk in our factories. These are given by Kṛṣṇa. So we should acknowledge this: "This food is given by Kṛṣṇa. Since it is Kṛṣṇa's, let me offer it first to Him. Then I will take the remnants as *prasādam.*" Everyone can do this, but people do not want to. They want to satisfy the tongue. But Kṛṣṇa forbids that in the *Bhagavad-gītā: bhuñjate te tv aghaṁ pāpāṁ ye pacanty ātma-kāraṇāt.* "One who cooks for himself eats only sin." If one is simply eating sin, how can he be happy? He will have to suffer. So, a devotee cooks only for Kṛṣṇa. A nondevotee thinks, "Look at this meat and chicken, bread and liquor. I will eat voraciously." Because he is eating nothing but sin, he will have to suffer.

Without Kṛṣṇa consciousness, everyone must suffer. That is the law of nature. As Kṛṣṇa says in the *Bhagavad-gītā*, *daivī hy eṣā guṇamayī mama māyā duratyayā:* "On your own you cannot avoid suffering the pains caused by my material nature." But, *mām eva ye prapadyante māyām etāṁ taranti te:* "You can be happy and free of suffering if you surrender to Me." That is the only way.

So, we have a propensity to love, but we do not know how to love or where our loving propensity should be reposed so that we and everyone else will be happy. The proper object of love is revealed in the *Śrīmad-Bhāgavatam* [4.31.14]:

yathā taror mūla-niṣecanena
tṛpyanti tat-skandha-bhujopaśākhāḥ
prāṇopahārāc ca yathendriyāṇāṁ
tathaiva sarvārhaṇam acyutejyā

"If you water the root of tree, the water is distributed to the branches, leaves, twigs, fruits, flowers—everywhere. Or, if you put food into the stomach, the energy is distributed all over the body. Similarly, if you love Kṛṣṇa, then everyone becomes satisfied."

Kṛṣṇa is the root of all existence (*ahaṁ sarvasya*

prabhavaḥ, janmādy asya yataḥ). But we are neglecting to water the root. Instead we are pouring water on the leaves and branches. But the leaves and branches are drying up, and we are becoming frustrated. In other words, so-called humanitarian service or social service without any touch of Kṛṣṇa consciousness is just like watering the leaves and branches of a tree without watering the root: it is all useless labor (*śrama eva hi kevalam*). You may perform whatever loving service you can for your society, community, and nation, but you must do it in Kṛṣṇa consciousness, for Kṛṣṇa's pleasure. Then your loving service will be perfect. Otherwise it will remain imperfect. The persons whom you are serving will never be happy, nor will you be happy.

So our ability to love one another will remain imperfectly fulfilled until we know who is the supreme beloved. The supreme beloved is Kṛṣṇa, the Supreme Person. He is supremely beautiful, supremely rich, supremely famous, supremely wise, supremely powerful, and supremely renounced—everything supreme. If someone has any of these six opulences, we love him. If one is very rich and charitable, for example, he is loved. Now, just think how rich and charitable Kṛṣṇa is! He is distributing food to millions and millions of living entities every day. We are proud if we can feed one hundred, two hundred, five hundred, two thousand people. But there are millions and millions of animals all over the world, and Kṛṣṇa is supplying them all with food. Actually, there is no scarcity of food. Human beings sometimes experience a scarcity of food because they misuse their advanced consciousness. Therefore they are put into trouble. If people would take up Kṛṣṇa consciousness, all these troubles would be finished.

The mission of our Kṛṣṇa consciousness movement is to teach people how to love Kṛṣṇa. Only then will they be fully satisfied. As it is said in the *Śrīmad-Bhāgavatam* [1.2.6]:

sa vai puṁsāṁ paro dharmo yato bhaktir adhokṣaje
ahaituky apratihatā yayātmā suprasīdati

"The supreme occupation for all humanity is that which awakens loving devotional service to Kṛṣṇa. When such devotional service is uninterrupted and free of selfish motives, it completely satisfies the self." Teaching this truth is the mission of the Kṛṣṇa consciousness movement. If people will accept it, all their problems will be solved, and they will be happy

Thank you very much.

Placing Our Love in Kṛṣṇa

In this talk Śrīla Prabhupāda says, "To love your home, to love your country, to love your husband, to love your children, to love your wife, and on and on—all this love is more or less present in the animal kingdom. But that sort of love will not give you happiness. You'll be frustrated. . . . If you really want peace, if you really want satisfaction, . . . then try to love Kṛṣṇa." (September 1968, Seattle, Washington)

Govindam ādi-puruṣaṁ tam ahaṁ bhajāmi. Our program is to worship Govinda, the original person, with love and devotion. This is Kṛṣṇa consciousness. We are teaching people to love Kṛṣṇa. That's all. Our program is to direct your love toward the proper place. Everyone wants to love, but they're being frustrated because their love is being misplaced. People do not understand where to place their love. First of all you love your body. Then, a little extended, you love your father and mother. Then you love your community, then your country, then the whole human society. And at last you love all living entities. But all this extended love will not give you satisfaction—until you reach the point of loving Kṛṣṇa. Then you'll be satisfied.

For example, when you throw a stone into a lake, a circle begins expanding. The circle keeps expanding, expanding, expanding . . . And when the circle touches the shore, it stops. Until the circle reaches the shore of the lake, it must go on increasing. So we have to go on increasing and increasing our love until we love Kṛṣṇa, the Supreme Personality of Godhead.

There are two ways to increase your love. You can practice loving your society, loving your country, loving all humanity, all living entities, and on and on. Or you can directly love Kṛṣṇa. Then everything is complete. It is so nice. Because Kṛṣṇa is all-attractive, love for Him includes everything. Why? Because Kṛṣṇa is the center of everything. In a family, if you love your father, then you love your brothers, your sisters, the servant of your father, the home of your father, the wife of your father (namely, your mother)—everyone. The central point is the father. Similarly, if you love Kṛṣṇa, then your love will be expanded everywhere.

Another example: If you love a tree, you can simply pour water on the root. Then the leaves, the flowers, the branches, the trunk, the twigs—everything—will be nourished. Then your love for the tree will be properly expressed. Similarly, if you love your countrymen, if you want to see that they become educated, advanced economically and mentally and physically, then what do you do? You pay taxes to the government; you don't hide your income tax. You simply pay taxes to the central government, and your money will be distributed to the education department, to the defense department, to the hygiene department—everywhere.

These are crude examples, but they show that if you actually want to love everyone and everything, you should love Kṛṣṇa. You'll not be frustrated, because loving Kṛṣṇa is complete. When your love is complete, you'll be completely satisfied. It is just like when you eat food to your full satisfaction: you say, "I am satisfied; I don't want any more."

So, this Kṛṣṇa consciousness movement is very simple. Although it was inaugurated five hundred years ago by Lord Caitanya Mahāprabhu, it is even older than that, since it is spoken of in the Vedic scriptures. From the historical point of view, this Kṛṣṇa consciousness movement has existed at least since Lord Kṛṣṇa appeared on the surface of this planet five thousand years ago. And more recently, five hundred years ago, Lord Caitanya expanded the movement. His mission is *ārādhyo bhagavān,* to propagate the worship of Bhagavān, the Supreme Personality of Godhead.

Everyone is subordinate to someone else. Everyone wants to be independent, but this is impossible. Nobody is independent; everyone is subordinate. Nobody can say, "I am completely independent." Is there anyone who can say this? No. Everyone is subordinate. And when you love someone, you willingly become subordinate. A girl says to a boy, "I want to become your subordinate." Why? That is our nature. We want to be subordinate, because our nature is to be subordinate. But we do not know to whom we should be subordinate so that we will become completely satisfied. We reject one subordination and accept another subordination. For example, a worker becomes subordinate to his boss because the boss gives him wages, say six hundred dollars monthly. Therefore the worker must worship the boss; the worker must please him. And if the worker finds some better wages in another place, he goes there. But that does not mean he becomes independent. He's still subordinate.

So, Lord Caitanya teaches that since you must be subordinate to somebody, since you must worship somebody, you should worship Kṛṣṇa. Then you'll be fully satisfied.

Then, *tad-dhāma vṛndāvanam.* If you want to worship somebody, then worship Kṛṣṇa, love Kṛṣṇa. And if you want to worship some place, worship His place, Vṛndāvana. Everyone wants to love some place—some country or nation. Somebody says, "I love this American land." Somebody says, "I love this Chinese land." Somebody says, "I love this Russian land." This is nationalism, *bhauma-ijya-dhīḥ.* A person is naturally inclined to love some material land, generally where he's born. So Caitanya Mahāprabhu says that because you are inclined to love some person, love Kṛṣṇa, and because you want to love some land, love Vṛndāvana. *Ārādhyo bhagavān vrajeśa-tanayas tad-dhāma vṛndāvanam.*

But suppose someone says, "I can't see Kṛṣṇa. How can I love Him?" Caitanya Mahāprabhu answers, *ramyā kācid upāsanā vrajavadhū-vargeṇa yā kalpitā.* If you want to learn the process of worshiping Kṛṣṇa, of loving Kṛṣṇa, just try to follow in the footsteps of the *gopīs,* the cowherd girls of Vṛndāvana. The *gopīs'* love for Kṛṣṇa is the highest perfectional love of God. There are different kinds of worship of God. The beginning is "O God, give us our daily bread." This is the beginning. When we are taught to worship God, we are instructed, "Go to church and pray to God for your necessities." But although that is the beginning, that is not pure love. Pure love for God can be found among the *gopīs*. Here is how they loved Kṛṣṇa:

Kṛṣṇa was a cowherd boy. With His friends, the other cowherd boys, He used to go with His cows to the pasturing ground for the whole day. (At that time people were satisfied with land and cows. That's all. That was the means of solving all economic problems. They did not work in big industries; they were not the servants of anyone. They simply took the production from the land and the milk from the cows, and their whole food problem was solved.) So, Kṛṣṇa used to go to the pasturing ground, and the *gopīs* stayed at home. Kṛṣṇa was miles away, in the pasturing ground, and the *gopīs* at home were thinking, "Oh, Kṛṣṇa's feet are so soft! Now He's walking on the rough ground, and the sharp pebbles are pricking His soles. So He must be feeling some pain." Thinking in this way, the *gopīs* used to cry. Just see. This is love.

When Kṛṣṇa returned they did not ask Him, "My dear Kṛṣṇa, what have You brought us from Your pasturing ground? What is in Your pocket? Let us see." No. They were simply thinking of how Kṛṣṇa could be satisfied. The *gopīs* used to dress themselves very nicely and go before Kṛṣṇa. While dressing they would think, "Oh, He'll be happy to see me." Generally, a boy or a man becomes happy to see his lover or wife nicely dressed. Therefore it is the nature of a woman to dress nicely just to satisfy her husband. If her husband is not at home, then she should not dress nicely. Women dress differently according to their positions, and by seeing a woman's dress one can immediately understand what she is. One can understand by seeing the dress that she is an unmarried girl, a married girl, a widow, or a prostitute. Dressing is so important.

So, we are not going to discuss the social customs of India. We are discussing the loving affairs of Kṛṣṇa and the *gopīs*. Their relationship was so intimate and so unalloyed that Kṛṣṇa Himself admitted, "My dear *gopīs,* it is not in My power to repay you for your love." Kṛṣṇa is the Supreme Personality of Godhead, yet He became bankrupt—He could not repay His debt to the *gopīs*. So the *gopīs* possessed the highest perfection of love for Kṛṣṇa.

I am describing the mission of Lord Caitanya. He is instructing us that the only lovable object is Kṛṣṇa, the only lovable land is Vṛndāvana, and the process of loving Kṛṣṇa is shown by the vivid example of the *gopīs*. There are different stages of devotees, and the *gopīs* are on the highest platform. And among the *gopīs*, the supreme is Rādhārāṇī. Therefore, nobody can surpass Rādhārāṇī's love for Kṛṣṇa.

Now, to learn this science of loving God, there must be some book, some authoritative literature. Yes, Caitanya Mahāprabhu says, that book is *Śrīmad-Bhāgavatam*. *Śrīmad-bhāgavatam pramāṇam amalam*. *Śrīmad-Bhāgavatam* is the spotless description of how to love God. There is no better description. From the beginning it teaches how to love God.

Those who have studied *Śrīmad-Bhāgavatam* know that the first verse in the First Canto is *janmādy asya yataḥ . . . satyaṁ paraṁ dhīmahi*. In the beginning the author says, "I am offering my unalloyed devotion unto the Supreme, from whom everything has emanated." So, it is a great description. If you want to learn how to love God, or Kṛṣṇa, then study *Śrīmad-Bhāgavatam*. And for understanding *Śrīmad-Bhāgavatam,* the preliminary study is *Bhagavad-gītā*. Study *Bhagavad-gītā* to understand the real nature or identity of God and yourself, and also to understand your relationship with God, and then when you are a little advanced, when you are fully convinced that Kṛṣṇa is the only lovable object, then the next book you should study is *Śrīmad-Bhāgavatam*.

Knowledge of the *Bhagavad-gītā As It Is* is the entrance examination. Just as students pass their high-school examination and then enter college, so you must pass your "high-school examination" in how to love God by studying *Bhagavad-gītā As It Is*. Then you should study *Śrīmad-Bhāgavatam*—that is the graduate course. And when you're still further advanced, on the postgraduate level, you should study *Śrī Caitanya-caritāmṛta*. So there is no difficulty in learning the science of loving Kṛṣṇa.

The fact is that we have to learn how to love Kṛṣṇa. The instruction is there and the method is there, and we are trying to serve you as far as possible. We are sending our boys into the streets to invite you, and if you kindly take up this opportunity, then your life will be successful. *Premā pum-artho mahān*. This human form of life is meant for developing love for God. In all other forms of life, we have loved something else—as birds we have loved our nests, as bees we have loved our hives, and so on. There is no necessity of teaching a bird or a bee how to love its offspring, because that is natural. To love your home, to love your country, to love your husband, to love your children, to love your wife, and on and on—all this love is more or less present in the animal kingdom. But that sort of love will not give you happiness. You'll be frustrated. Because the body is temporary, all these loving affairs are also temporary. And they're not pure; they are simply a perverted reflection of the pure love existing between you and Kṛṣṇa. So if you really want peace, if you really want satisfaction, if you don't want to be confused, then try to love Kṛṣṇa. Then your life will be successful.

The Kṛṣṇa consciousness movement is not something manufactured to mislead or bluff people. It is the most authorized movement, based on the Vedic literature—the *Bhagavad-gītā*, *Śrīmad-Bhāgavatam*, *Caitanya-caritāmṛta*, and other scriptures—and many, many great saintly persons have adopted the process of Kṛṣṇa consciousness as the means of attaining perfection. The vivid example is Lord Caitanya. You see that in His picture He is chanting and dancing in ecstasy. So you have to learn this art; then your life will be successful. You don't have to practice something artificial and speculate and bother your brain and so on. You have the instinct for loving others; it is natural. You are simply misplacing your love, and therefore you are frustrated and confused. So if you don't want to be confused, if you don't want to be frustrated, then try to love Kṛṣṇa. You will feel how you are making progress in peace, in happiness, in everything that you want.

Thank you very much.

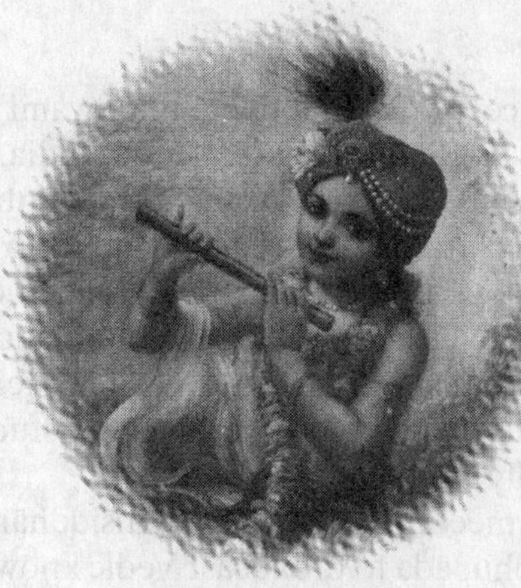

Appendixes

About the Author

His Divine Grace A. C. Bhaktivedanta Swami Prabhupāda appeared in this world in 1896 in Calcutta, India. He first met his spiritual master, Śrīla Bhaktisiddhānta Sarasvatī Gosvāmī, in Calcutta in 1922. Bhaktisiddhānta Sarasvatī, a prominent religious scholar and the founder of sixty-four Gauḍīya Maṭhas (Vedic institutes), liked this educated young man and convinced him to dedicate his life to teaching Vedic knowledge. Śrīla Prabhupāda became his student and, in 1932, his formally initiated disciple.

At their first meeting, in 1922, Bhaktisiddhānta Sarasvatī asked Śrīla Prabhupāda to broadcast Vedic knowledge in English. In the years that followed, Śrīla Prabhupāda wrote a commentary on the *Bhagavad-gītā,* assisted the Gauḍīya Maṭha in its work, and, in 1944, started *Back to Godhead,* an English fortnightly magazine. Single-handedly, Śrīla Prabhupāda edited it, typed the manuscripts, checked the galley proofs, and even distributed the individual copies. The magazine is now being continued by his disciples in the West.

In 1950 Śrīla Prabhupāda retired from married life, adopting the *vānaprastha* (retired) order to devote more time to his studies and writing. He traveled to the holy city of Vṛndāvana, where he lived in humble circumstances in the historic temple of Rādhā-Dāmodara. There he engaged for several years in deep study and writing. He accepted the renounced order of life (*sannyāsa*) in 1959. At Rādhā-Dāmodara, Śrīla Prabhupāda began work on his life's masterpiece: a multivolume commentated translation of the eighteen-thousand-verse *Śrīmad-Bhāgavatam* (*Bhāgavata Purāṇa*). He also wrote *Easy Journey to Other Planets.*

After publishing three volumes of the *Bhāgavatam,* Śrīla Prabhupāda came to the United States, in September 1965, to fulfill the mission of his spiritual master. Subsequently, His Divine Grace wrote more than fifty volumes of authoritative commentated translations and summary studies of the philosophical and religious classics of India.

When he first arrived in New York City, Śrīla Prabhupāda was nearly penniless. Only after a year of great difficulty did he establish the International Society for Krishna Consciousness, in July of 1966. Before he passed away on November 14, 1977, he had guided the Society and seen it grow to a worldwide confederation of more than one hundred *āśramas,* schools, temples, institutes, and farm communities.

In 1972 His Divine Grace introduced the Vedic system of primary and secondary education in the West by founding the *gurukula* school in Dallas, Texas. Since then his disciples have established similar schools throughout the United States and the rest of the world.

Śrīla Prabhupāda also inspired the construction of several large international cultural centers in India. The center at Śrīdhāma Māyāpur is the site for a planned spiritual city, an ambitions project for which construction will extend over many years to come. In Vṛndāvana are the magnificent Kṛṣṇa-Balarāma Temple and International Guesthouse, *gurukula* school, and Śrīla Prabhupāda Memorial and Museum. There are also major cultural and educational centers in Mumbai, New Delhi, and Bangalore. Other centers are either underway or planned in a dozen important locations on the Indian subcontinent.

Śrīla Prabhupāda's most significant contribution, however, is his books. Highly respected by scholars for their authority, depth, and clarity, they are used as textbooks in numerous college courses. His writings have been translated into over fifty languages. The Bhaktivedanta Book Trust, established in 1972 to publish the works of His Divine Grace, has thus become the world's largest publisher of books in the field of Indian religion and philosophy.

In just twelve years, in spite of his advanced age, Śrīla Prabhupāda circled the globe fourteen times on lecture tours that took him to six continents. In spite of such a vigorous schedule, Śrīla Prabhupāda continued to write prolifically. His writings constitute a veritable library of Vedic philosophy, religion, literature, and culture.

An Introduction to ISKCON And Devotee Lifestyle

What Is ISKCON?

The International Society for Krishna Consciousness (ISKCON), popularly known as the Hare Kṛṣṇa movement, is a worldwide association of devotees of Kṛṣṇa, the Supreme Personality of Godhead. God is known by many names, according to His different qualities and activities. In the Bible he is known as Jehovah ("the almighty one"), in the Koran as Allah ("the great one"), and in the *Bhagavad-gītā* as Kṛṣṇa, a Sanskrit name meaning "the all-attractive one."

The movement's main purpose is to promote the well-being of human society by teaching the science of God consciousness (Kṛṣṇa consciousness) according to the timeless Vedic scriptures of India.

Many leading figures in the international religious and academic community have affirmed the movement's authenticity. Diana L. Eck, professor of comparative religion and Indiań studies at Harvard University, describes the movement as "a tradition that commands a respected place in the religious life of humankind."

In 1965, His Divine Grace A. C. Bhaktivedanta Swami, known to his followers as Śrīla Prabhupāda, brought Kṛṣṇa consciousness to America. On the day he landed in Boston, on his way to New York City, he penned these words in his diary: "My dear Lord Kṛṣṇa, I am sure that when this transcendental message penetrates [the hearts of the Westerners], they will certainly feel gladdened and thus become liberated from all unhappy conditions of life." He was sixty-nine years old, alone and with few resources, but the wealth of spiritual knowledge and devotion he possessed was an unwavering source of strength and inspiration.

"At a very advanced age, when most people would be resting on their laurels," writes Harvey Cox, Harvard University theologian and author, "Śrīla Prabhupāda harkened to the mandate of his own spiritual teacher and set out on the difficult and demanding voyage to America. Śrīla Prabhupāda is, of course, only one of thousands of teachers. But in another sense, he is one in a thousand, maybe one in a million."

In 1966, Śrīla Prabhupāda founded the International Society for Krishna Consciousness, which became the formal name for the Hare Kṛṣṇa movement.

Astonishing Growth

In the years that followed, Śrīla Prabhupāda gradually attracted tens of thousands of followers, started more than a hundred temples and ashrams, and published scores of books. His achievement is remarkable in that he transplanted India's ancient spiritual culture to the twentieth-century Western world.

New devotees of Kṛṣṇa soon became highly visible in all the major cities around the world by their public chanting and their distribution of Śrīla Prabhupāda's books of Vedic knowledge. They began staging joyous cultural festivals throughout the year and serving millions of plates of delicious vegetarian food offered to Kṛṣṇa (known as *prasādam*). As a result, ISKCON has significantly influenced the lives of millions of people. In the early 1980's the late A. L. Basham, one of the world's leading authorities on Indian history and culture, wrote, "The Hare Kṛṣṇa movement arose out of next to nothing in less than twenty years and has become known all over the West. This is an important fact in the history of the Western world."

Five Thousand Years of Spiritual Wisdom

Scholars worldwide have acclaimed Śrīla Prabhupāda's translations of Vedic literature. Garry Gelade, a professor at Oxford University's Department of Philosophy, wrote of them:

"These texts are to be treasured. No one of whatever faith or philosophical persuasion who reads these books with an open mind can fail to be moved and impressed." And Dr. Larry Shinn, Dean of the College of Arts and Sciences at Bucknell University, wrote, "Prabhupāda's personal piety gave him real authority. He exhibited complete command of the scriptures, an unusual depth of realization, and an outstanding personal example, because he actually lived what he taught."

The best known of the Vedic texts, the *Bhagavad-gītā* ("Song of God"), is the philosophical basis for the Hare Kṛṣṇa movement. Dating back 5,000 years, it is sacred to nearly a billion people today. This exalted work has been praised by scholars and leaders the world over. Mahatma Gandhi said, "When doubts haunt me, when disappointments stare me in the face and I see not one ray of hope, I turn to the *Bhagavad-gītā* and find a verse to comfort me." Ralph Waldo Emerson wrote, "It was the first of books; it was as if an empire spoke to us, nothing small or unworthy, but large, serene, consistent, the voice of an old intelligence which in another age and climate had pondered and thus disposed of the same questions which exercise us." It is not surprising to anyone familiar with the *Gītā* that Henry David Thoreau said, "In the morning I bathe my intellect in the stupendous and cosmogonal philosophy of the *Bhagavad-gītā*."

As Dr. Shinn pointed out, Śrīla Prabhupāda's *Bhagavad-gītā* (titled *Bhagavad-gītā As It Is*) possesses unique authority not only because of his erudition but because he lived what he taught. Thus unlike the many other English translations of the *Gītā* that preceded his, which is replete with extensive commentary, Śrīla Prabhupāda's has sparked a spiritual revolution throughout the world.

Lord Kṛṣṇa teaches in the *Bhagavad-gītā* that we are not these temporary material bodies but spirit souls, or conscious entities, and that we can find genuine peace and happiness only in spiritual devotion to Him, the Supreme Personality of Godhead.

A Sixteenth-Century Incarnation of Kṛṣṇa

Lord Śrī Caitanya Mahāprabhu, a sixteenth-century full incarnation of Kṛṣṇa, popularized the chanting of God's names all over India. He constantly sang these names of God, as prescribed in the Vedic literatures: Hare Kṛṣṇa, Hare Kṛṣṇa, Kṛṣṇa Kṛṣṇa, Hare Hare/ Hare Rāma, Hare Rāma, Rāma Rāma, Hare Hare. This Hare Kṛṣṇa chant, or *mantra,* is a transcendental sound vibration. It purifies the mind and awakens the dormant love of God that resides in the hearts of all living beings. Lord Caitanya requested His followers to spread the chanting to every town and village of the world.

Anyone can take part in the chanting of Hare Kṛṣṇa and learn the science of spiritual devotion by studying the *Bhagavad-gītā As It Is*. This easy and practical process of self-realization will awaken our natural state of peace and happiness.

Hare Kṛṣṇa Lifestyles

The devotees seen dancing and chanting in the streets, dressed in traditional Indian robes, are for the most part full-time students of the Hare Kṛṣṇa movement. The vast majority of followers, however, live and work in the general community, practicing Kṛṣṇa consciousness in their homes and attending temples on a regular basis.

Full-time devotees throughout the world number about 15,000, with 500,000 congregational members. The movement comprises 300 temples, 50 rural communities, 40 schools, and 75 restaurants in 85 countries.

In order to revive their own and humanity's inherent natural spiritual principles of compassion, truthfulness, cleanliness, and austerity, and to master the mind and the material senses, devotees also follow these four regulations (please see page 254 for an explanation):

1. No eating of meat, fish, or eggs.
2. No gambling.
3. No illicit sex.

4. No intoxication of any kind, including tobacco, coffee, and tea.

According to the *Bhagavad-gītā* and other Vedic literatures, indulgence in the above activities disrupts our physical, mental, and spiritual well-being and increases anxiety and conflict in society.

A Philosophy for Everyone

The philosophy of the Hare Kṛṣṇa movement (a monotheistic tradition) is summarized in the following eight points:

1. By sincerely cultivating the authentic spiritual science presented in the *Bhagavad-gītā* and other Vedic scriptures, we can become free from anxiety and achieve a state of pure, unending, blissful consciousness.

2. Each of us is not the material body but an eternal spirit soul, part and parcel of God (Kṛṣṇa). As such, we are all the eternal servants of Kṛṣṇa and are interrelated through Him, our common father.

3. Kṛṣṇa is the eternal, all-knowing, omnipresent, all-powerful, and all-attractive Personality of Godhead. He is the seed-giving father of all living beings and the sustaining energy of the universe. He is the source of all incarnations of God, including Lord Buddha and Lord Jesus Christ.

4. The *Vedas* are the oldest scriptures in the world. The essence of the *Vedas* is found in the *Bhagavad-gītā,* a literal record of Kṛṣṇa's words spoken five thousands years ago in India. The goal of Vedic knowledge—and of all religions—is to achieve love of God.

5. We can perfectly understand the knowledge of self-realization through the instructions of a genuine spiritual master—one who is free from selfish motives, who teaches the science of God explained in the *Bhagavad-gītā,* and whose mind is firmly fixed in meditation on Kṛṣṇa.

6. All that we eat should first be offered to Lord Kṛṣṇa with a prayer. In this way Kṛṣṇa accepts the offering and blesses it for our purification.

7. Rather than living in a self-centered way, we should act for the pleasure of Lord Kṛṣṇa. This is known as *bhakti-yoga,* the science of devotional service.

8. The most effective means for achieving God consciousness in this Age of Kali, or quarrel, is to chant the holy names of the Lord: Hare Kṛṣṇa, Hare Kṛṣṇa, Kṛṣṇa Kṛṣṇa, Hare Hare/ Hare Rāma, Hare Rāma, Rāma Rāma, Hare Hare.

Kṛṣṇa Consciousness at Home

by Mahātmā dāsa

In *The Quest for Enlightenment* Śrīla Prabhupāda makes it clear how important it is for everyone to practice Kṛṣṇa consciousness, devotional service to Lord Kṛṣṇa. Of course, living in the association of Kṛṣṇa's devotees in a temple or *āśrama* makes it easier to practice devotional service. But if you're determined, you can follow at home the teachings of Kṛṣṇa consciousness and thus convert your home into a temple.

Spiritual life, like material life, means practical activity. The difference is that whereas we perform material activities for the benefit of ourselves or those we consider ours, we perform spiritual activities for the benefit of Lord Kṛṣṇa, under the guidance of the scriptures and the spiritual master. The key is to accept the guidance of the scripture and the guru. Kṛṣṇa declares in the *Bhagavad-gītā* that a person can achieve neither happiness nor the supreme destination of life—going back to Godhead, back to Lord Kṛṣṇa—if he or she does not follow the injunctions of the scriptures. And *how* to follow the scriptural rules by engaging in practical service to the Lord—that is explained by a bona fide spiritual master. Without following the instructions of a spiritual master who is in an authorized chain of disciplic succession coming from Kṛṣṇa Himself, we cannot make spiritual progress. The practices outlined here are the timeless practices of *bhakti-yoga* as given by the foremost spiritual master and exponent of Kṛṣṇa consciousness in our time, His Divine Grace A. C. Bhaktivedanta Swami Prabhupāda, founder-*ācārya* of the International Society for Krishna Consciousness (ISKCON).

The purpose of spiritual knowledge is to bring us closer to God, or Kṛṣṇa. Kṛṣṇa says in the *Bhagavad-gītā* (18.55), *bhaktyā māṁ abhijānāti:* "I can be known only by devotional service." Knowledge guides us in proper action. Spiritual knowledge directs us to satisfy the desires of Kṛṣṇa through practical engagements in His loving service. Without practical application, theoretical knowledge is of little value.

Spiritual knowledge is meant to direct us in all aspects of life. We should endeavor, therefore, to organize our lives in such a way as to follow Kṛṣṇa's teachings as far as possible. We should try to do our best, to do more than is simply convenient. Then it will be possible for us to rise to the transcendental plane of Kṛṣṇa consciousness, even while living far from a temple.

Chanting the Hare Kṛṣṇa Mantra

The first principle in devotional service is to chant the Hare Kṛṣṇa *mahā-mantra* (*mahā* means "great"; *mantra* means "sound that liberates the mind from ignorance"):

Hare Kṛṣṇa, Hare Kṛṣṇa, Kṛṣṇa Kṛṣṇa, Hare Hare
Hare Rāma, Hare Rāma, Rāma Rāma, Hare Hare

You can chant these holy names of the Lord anywhere and at any time, but it is best to set a specific time of the day to regularly chant. Early morning hours are ideal.

The chanting can be done in two ways: singing the *mantra,* called *kīrtana* (usually done in a group), and saying the *mantra* to oneself, called *japa* (which literally means "to speak softly"). Concentrate on hearing the sound of the holy names. As you chant, pronounce the names clearly and distinctly, addressing Kṛṣṇa in a prayerful mood. When your mind wanders, bring it back to the sound of the Lord's names. Chanting is a prayer to Kṛṣṇa that means "O energy of the Lord [Hare], O all-attractive Lord [Kṛṣṇa], O Supreme Enjoyer [Rāma], please engage me in Your service." The more attentively and sincerely you chant these names of God, the more spiritual progress you will make.

Since God is all-powerful and all-merciful, He has kindly made it very easy for us to chant His names, and He has also invested all His powers in them. Therefore the names of God and God Himself are identical. This means that when we chant the holy names of Kṛṣṇa and Rāma we are directly associating with God and being purified. Therefore we should always try to chant with devotion and reverence. The Vedic literature states that Lord Kṛṣṇa is personally dancing on your tongue when you chant His holy name.

When you chant alone, it is best to chant on *japa* beads (provided in the Mantra Meditation Kit, which is available in the advertisement section at the end of this book). This not only helps you fix your attention on the holy name, but it also helps you count the number of times you chant the *mantra* daily. Each strand of *japa* beads contains 108 small beads and one large bead, the head bead. Begin on a bead next to the head bead and gently roll it between the thumb and middle finger of your right hand as you chant the full Hare Kṛṣṇa *mantra.* Then move to the next bead and repeat the process. In this way, chant on each of the 108 beads until you reach the head bead again. This is one round of *japa*. Then, without chanting on the head bead, reverse the beads and

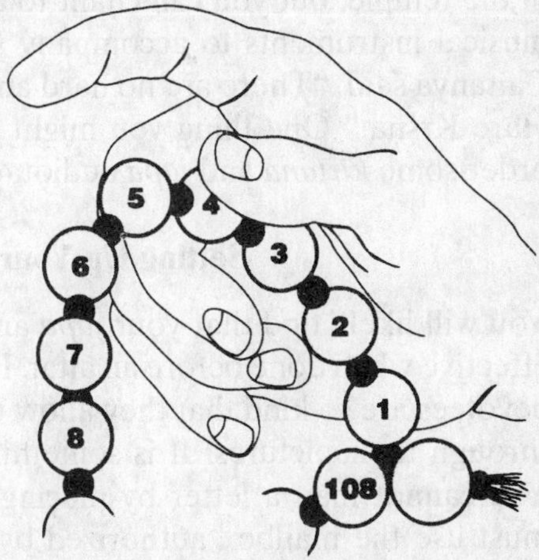

start your second round on the last bead you chanted on.

Initiated devotees vow before the spiritual master to chant at least sixteen rounds of the Hare Kṛṣṇa *mantra* daily. But even if you can chant only one round a day, the principle is that once you commit yourself to chanting that round, you should try complete it every day without fail. When you feel you can chant more, then increase the minimum number of rounds you chant each day—but don't fall below that number. You can chant more than your fixed number, but you should maintain a set minimum each day. (Please note that the beads are sacred and therefore should never touch the ground or be put in an unclean place. To keep your beads clean, it's best to carry them in a special bead bag, such as the one that comes as part of the Mantra Meditation Kit.)

Aside from chanting *japa,* you can also sing the Lord's holy names in *kīrtana*. While you can perform *kīrtana* individually, it is generally performed with others. A melodious *kīrtana* with family or friends is sure to enliven everyone. ISKCON devotees use traditional melodies and instruments, especially in the temple, but you can chant to any melody and use any musical instruments to accompany your chanting. As Lord Caitanya said, "There are no hard and fast rules for chanting Hare Kṛṣṇa." One thing you might want to do, however, is order some *kīrtana* and *japa* audiotapes (see ads).

Setting Up Your Altar

You will likely find that your *japa* and *kīrtana* are especially effective when done before an altar. Lord Kṛṣṇa and His pure devotees are so kind that they allow us to worship them even through their pictures. It is something like mailing a letter: You cannot mail a letter by placing it in just any box; you must use the mailbox authorized by the government. Similarly, we cannot imagine a picture of God and worship that, but we can worship the authorized picture of God, and Kṛṣṇa accepts our worship through that picture.

Setting up an altar at home means receiving the Lord and

His pure devotees as your most honored guests. Where should you set up the altar? Well, how would you seat a guest? An ideal place would be clean, well lit, and free from drafts and household disturbances. Your guest, of course, would need a comfortable chair, but for the picture of Kṛṣṇa's form a wall shelf, a mantelpiece, a corner table, or the top shelf of a bookcase will do. You wouldn't seat a guest in your home and then ignore him; you'd provide a place for yourself to sit, too, where you could comfortably face him and enjoy his company. So don't make your altar inaccessible.

What do you need for an altar? Here are the essentials:

1. A picture of Śrīla Prabhupāda.
2. A picture of Lord Caitanya and His associates.
3. A picture of Śrī Śrī Rādhā-Kṛṣṇa.

In addition, you may want an altar cloth, water cups (one for each picture), candles with holders, a special plate for offering food, a small bell, incense, an incense holder, and fresh flowers, which you may offer in vases or simply place before each picture. If you're interested in more elaborate Deity worship, ask any of the ISKCON devotees or write to BBT (see order form in the back of this book).

The first person we worship on the altar is the spiritual master. The spiritual master is not God. Only God is God.

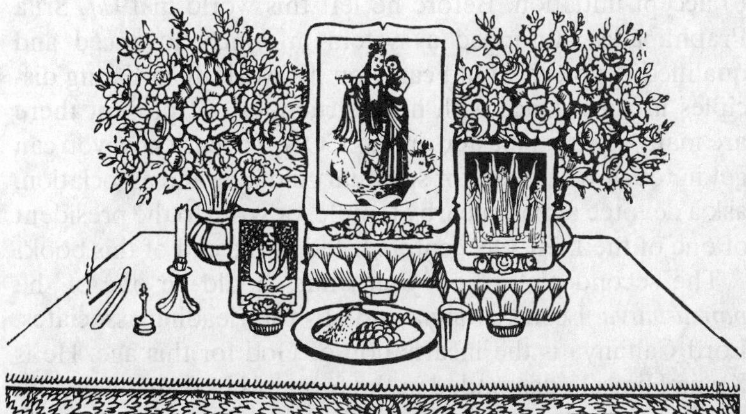

But because the spiritual master is His dearmost servant, God has empowered him, and therefore he deserves the same respect as that given to God. He links the disciple with God and teaches him the process of *bhakti-yoga.* He is God's ambassador to the material world. When a president sends an ambassador to a foreign country, the ambassador receives the same respect as that accorded the president, and the ambassador's words are as authoritative as the president's. Similarly, we should respect the spiritual master as we would God, and revere his words as we would His.

There are two main kinds of *gurus:* the instructing *guru* and the initiating *guru.* Everyone who takes up the process of *bhakti-yoga* as a result of coming in contact with ISKCON owes an immense debt of gratitude to Śrīla Prabhupāda. Before Śrīla Prabhupāda left India in 1965 to spread Kṛṣṇa consciousness abroad, almost no one outside India knew anything about the practice of pure devotional service to Lord Kṛṣṇa. Therefore, everyone who has learned of the process through his books, his *Back to Godhead* magazine, his tapes, or contact with his followers should offer respect to Śrīla Prabhupāda. As the founder and spiritual guide of the International Society for Krishna Consciousness, he is the instructing *guru* of us all.

As you progress in *bhakti-yoga,* you may eventually want to accept initiation. Before he left this world in 1977, Śrīla Prabhupāda authorized a system in which advanced and qualified devotees would carry on his work by initiating disciples in accordance with his instructions. At present there are many spiritual masters in ISKCON. To learn how you can get in touch with them for spiritual guidance and association, ask a devotee at your nearby temple, or write to the president of one of the ISKCON centers listed at the end of this book.

The second picture on your altar should be one of the *pañca-tattva,* Lord Caitanya and His four leading associates. Lord Caitanya is the incarnation of God for this age. He is Kṛṣṇa Himself, descended in the form of His own devotee to teach us how to surrender to Him, specifically by chanting

His holy names and performing other activities of *bhakti-yoga.* Lord Caitanya is the most merciful incarnation, for He makes it easy for anyone to attain love of God through the chanting of the Hare Kṛṣṇa *mantra.*

And of course your altar should have a picture of the Supreme Personality of Godhead, Lord Śrī Kṛṣṇa, with His eternal consort, Śrīmatī Rādhārāṇī. Śrīmatī Rādhārāṇī is Kṛṣṇa's spiritual potency. She is devotional service personified, and devotees always take shelter of Her to learn how to serve Kṛṣṇa.

You can arrange the pictures in a triangle, with the picture of Śrīla Prabhupāda on the left, the picture of Lord Caitanya and His associates on the right, and the picture of Rādhā and Kṛṣṇa, which, if possible, should be slightly larger than the others, on a small raised platform behind and in the center. Or you can hang the picture of Rādhā and Kṛṣṇa on the wall above.

Carefully clean the altar each morning. Cleanliness is essential in Deity worship. Remember, you wouldn't neglect to clean the room of an important guest, and when you establish an altar you invite Kṛṣṇa and His pure devotees to reside as the most exalted guests in your home. If you have water cups, rinse them out and fill them with fresh water daily. Then place them conveniently close to the pictures. You should remove flowers in vases as soon as they're slightly wilted, or daily if you've offered them at the base of the pictures. You should offer fresh incense at least once a day, and, if possible, light candles and place them near the pictures when you're chanting before the altar.

Please try the things we've suggested so far. It's very simple, really: If you try to love God, you'll gradually realize how much He loves you. That's the essence of *bhakti-yoga.*

Prasādam: How to Eat Spiritually

By His immense transcendental energies, Kṛṣṇa can actually convert matter into spirit. If we place an iron rod in a fire, before long the rod becomes red hot and acts just like fire. In the same way, food prepared for and offered to Kṛṣṇa with love and devotion becomes completely spiritualized. Such food is called Kṛṣṇa *prasādam,* which means "the mercy of Lord Kṛṣṇa."

Eating *prasādam* is a fundamental practice of *bhakti-yoga.* In other forms of yoga one must artificially repress the senses, but the *bhakti-yogī* can engage his or her senses in a variety of pleasing spiritual activities, such as tasting delicious food offered to Lord Kṛṣṇa. In this way the senses gradually become spiritualized and bring the devotee more and more transcendental pleasure by being engaged in devotional service. Such spiritual pleasure far surpasses any material experience.

Lord Caitanya said of *prasādam,* "Everyone has tasted these foods before. However, now that they have been prepared for Kṛṣṇa and offered to Him with devotion, these foods have acquired extraordinary tastes and uncommon fragrances. Just taste them and see the difference in the experience! Apart from the taste, even the fragrance pleases the mind and makes one forget any other fragrance. Therefore, it should be understood that the spiritual nectar of Kṛṣṇa's lips must have touched these ordinary foods and imparted to them all their transcendental qualities."

Eating only food offered to Kṛṣṇa is the perfection of vegetarianism. In itself, being a vegetarian is not enough; after all, even pigeons and monkeys are vegetarians. But when we go beyond vegetarianism to a diet of *prasādam,* our eating becomes helpful in achieving the goal of human life—reawakening the soul's original relationship with God. In the *Bhagavad-gītā* Lord Kṛṣṇa says that unless one eats only food that has been offered to Him in sacrifice, one will suffer the reactions of *karma.*

How to Prepare and Offer Prasādam

As you walk down the supermarket aisles selecting the foods

you will offer to Kṛṣṇa, you need to know what is offerable and what is not. In the *Bhagavad-gītā,* Lord Kṛṣṇa states, "If one offers Me with love and devotion a leaf, a flower, a fruit, or water, I will accept it." From this verse it is understood that we can offer Kṛṣṇa foods prepared from milk products, vegetables, fruits, nuts, and grains. (See the ads for one of the many Hare Kṛṣṇa cookbooks.) Meat, fish, and eggs are not offerable. And a few vegetarian items are also forbidden—garlic and onions, for example, which are in the mode of darkness. (*Hing,* or asafetida, is a tasty substitute for them in cooking and is available at most Indian groceries and ISKCON temple stores.) Nor can you offer to Kṛṣṇa coffee or tea that contain caffeine. If you like these beverages, purchase caffeine-free coffee and herbal teas.

While shopping, be aware that you may find meat, fish, and egg products mixed with other foods; so be sure to read labels carefully. For instance, some brands of yogurt and sour cream contain gelatin, a substance made from the horns, hooves, and bones of slaughtered animals. Also, make sure the cheese you buy contains no animal rennet, an enzyme extracted from the stomach tissues of slaughtered calves. Most hard cheese sold in America contains this rennet, so be careful about any cheese you can't verify as being free from animal rennet.

Also avoid foods cooked by nondevotees. According to the subtle laws of nature, the cook acts upon the food not only physically but mentally as well. Food thus becomes an agent for subtle influences on your consciousness. The principle is the same as that at work with a painting: a painting is not simply a collection of strokes on a canvas but an expression of the artist's state of mind, which affects the viewer. So if you eat food cooked by nondevotees—employees working in a factory, for example—then you're sure to absorb a dose of materialism and *karma*. So as far as possible use only fresh, natural ingredients.

In preparing food, cleanliness is the most important principle. Nothing impure should be offered to God; so keep your kitchen very clean. Always wash your hands thoroughly before entering the kitchen. While preparing food, do not taste it, for you are cooking the meal not for yourself but for the pleasure of Kṛṣṇa. Arrange portions of the food on dinnerware kept especially for this purpose; no one but the Lord should eat from these dishes. The easiest way to offer food is simply to pray, "My dear Lord Kṛṣṇa, please accept this food," and to chant each of the following prayers three times while ringing a bell (see the Sanskrit Pronunciation Guide on page 257):

1. Prayer to Śrīla Prabhupāda:

nama oṁ viṣṇu-pādāya kṛṣṇa-preṣṭhāya bhū-tale
śrīmate bhaktivedānta-svāminn iti nāmine

namas te sārasvate deve gaura-vāṇī-pracāriṇe
nirviśeṣa-śūnyavādi-pāścātya-deśa-tāriṇe

"I offer my respectful obeisances unto His Divine Grace A. C. Bhaktivedanta Swami Prabhupāda, who is very dear to Lord Kṛṣṇa, having taken shelter at His lotus feet. Our respectful obeisances are unto you, O spiritual master, servant of Bhaktisiddhānta Sarasvatī Gosvāmī. You are kindly preaching the message of Lord Caitanyadeva and delivering the Western countries, which are filled with impersonalism and voidism."

2. Prayer to Lord Caitanya:

namo mahā-vadānyāya kṛṣṇa-prema-pradāya te
kṛṣṇāya kṛṣṇa-caitanya-nāmne gaura-tviṣe namaḥ

"O most munificent incarnation! You are Kṛṣṇa Himself appearing as Śrī Kṛṣṇa Caitanya Mahāprabhu. You have assumed the golden color of Śrīmatī Rādhārāṇī, and You are widely distributing pure love of Kṛṣṇa. We offer our respectful obeisances unto You."

3. Prayer to Lord Kṛṣṇa:

namo brahmaṇya-devāya go-brāhmaṇa-hitāya ca
jagad-dhitāya kṛṣṇāya govindāya namo namaḥ

"I offer my respectful obeisances unto Lord Kṛṣṇa, who is the worshipable Deity for all *brāhmaṇas*, the well-wisher of the cows and the *brāhmaṇas,* and the benefactor of the whole world. I offer my repeated obeisances to the Personality of Godhead, known as Kṛṣṇa and Govinda."

Remember that the real purpose of preparing and offering food to the Lord is to show your devotion and gratitude to Him. Kṛṣṇa accepts your devotion, not the physical offering itself. God is complete in Himself—He doesn't need anything—but out of His immense kindness He allows us to offer food to Him so that we can develop our love for Him.

After offering the food to the Lord, wait at least five minutes for Him to partake of the preparations. Then you should transfer the food from the special dinnerware and wash the dishes and utensils you used for the offering. Now you and any guests may eat the *prasādam.* While you eat, try to appreciate the spiritual value of the food. Remember that because Kṛṣṇa has accepted it, it is nondifferent from Him, and therefore by eating it you will become purified.

Everything you offer on your altar becomes *prasādam,* the mercy of the Lord. Flowers, incense, the water, the food—everything you offer for the Lord's pleasure becomes spiritualized. The Lord enters into the offerings, and thus the remnants are nondifferent from Him. So you should not only deeply respect the things you've offered, but you should distribute them to others as well. Distribution of *prasādam* is an essential part of Deity worship.

Everyday Life: The Four Regulative Principles

Anyone serious about progressing in Kṛṣṇa consciousness must try to avoid the following four sinful activities:

1. Eating meat, fish, or eggs. These foods are saturated with the modes of passion and ignorance and therefore cannot be

offered to the Lord. A person who eats these foods participates in a conspiracy of violence against helpless animals and thus stops his spiritual progress dead in its tracks.

2. Gambling. Gambling invariably puts one into anxiety and fuels greed, envy, and anger.

3. The use of intoxicants. Drugs, alcohol, and tobacco, as well as any drinks or foods containing caffeine, cloud the mind, overstimulate the senses, and make it impossible to understand or follow the principles of *bhakti-yoga.*

4. Illicit sex. This is sex outside of marriage or sex in marriage for any purpose other than procreation. Sex for pleasure compels one to identify with the body and takes one far from Kṛṣṇa consciousness. The scriptures teach that sex is the most powerful force binding us to the material world. Anyone serious about advancing in Kṛṣṇa consciousness should minimize sex or eliminate it entirely.

Engagement in Practical Devotional Service

Everyone must do some kind of work, but if you work only for yourself you must accept the karmic reactions of that work. As Lord Kṛṣṇa says in the *Bhagavad-gītā* (3.9), "Work done as a sacrifice for Viṣṇu [Kṛṣṇa] has to be performed. Otherwise work binds one to the material world."

You needn't change your occupation, except if you're now engaged in a sinful job such as working as a butcher or bartender. If you're a writer, write for Kṛṣṇa; if you're an artist, create for Kṛṣṇa; if you're a secretary, type for Kṛṣṇa. You may also directly help the temple in your spare time, and you should sacrifice some of the fruits of your work by contributing a portion of your earnings to help maintain the temple and propagate Kṛṣṇa consciousness. Some devotees living outside the temple buy Hare Kṛṣṇa literature and distribute it to their friends and associates, or they engage in a variety of services at the temple. There is also a wide network of devotees who gather in each other's homes for chanting, worship, and study. Write to your local temple or the Society's secretary to learn of any such programs near you.

Additional Devotional Principles

There are many more devotional practices that can help you become Kṛṣṇa conscious. Here are two vital ones:

Studying Hare Kṛṣṇa literature. Śrīla Prabhupāda, the founder-*ācārya* of ISKCON, dedicated much of his time to writing books such as the *Bhagavad-gītā* and *Śrīmad-Bhāgavatam,* both of which are quoted extensively in *The Quest for Enlightenment*. Hearing the words—or reading the writings—of a realized spiritual master is an essential spiritual practice. So try to set aside some time every day to read Śrīla Prabhupāda's books. You can get a free catalog of available books and tapes from the BBT.

Associating with devotees. Śrīla Prabhupāda established the Hare Kṛṣṇa movement to give people in general the chance to associate with devotees of the Lord. This is the best way to gain faith in the process of Kṛṣṇa consciousness and become enthusiastic in devotional service. Conversely, maintaining intimate connections with nondevotees slows one's spiritual progress. So try to visit the Hare Kṛṣṇa center nearest you as often as possible.

In Closing

The beauty of Kṛṣṇa consciousness is that you can take as much as you're ready for. Kṛṣṇa Himself promises in the *Bhagavad-gītā* (2.40), "There is no loss or diminution in this endeavor, and even a little advancement on this path protects one from the most fearful type of danger." So bring Kṛṣṇa into your daily life, and we guarantee you'll feel the benefit.

Hare Kṛṣṇa!

Sanskrit Pronunciation Guide

The system of transliteration used in this book conforms to a system that scholars have accepted to indicate the pronunciation of each sound in the Sanskrit language.

The short vowel **a** is pronounced like the **u** in b**u**t, long **ā** like the **a** in f**a**r. Short **i** is pronounced as in p**i**n, long **ī** as in p**i**que, short **u** as in p**u**ll, and long **ū** as in r**u**le. The vowel **ṛ** is pronounced like the **ri** in **ri**m, **e** like the **ey** in th**ey**, **o** like the **o** in g**o, ai** like the **ai** in **ai**sle, and **au** like the **ow** in h**ow**. The *anusvāra* (**ṁ**) is pronounced like the **n** in the French word *bo***n**, and *visarga* (**ḥ**) is pronounced as a Þnal **h** sound. At the end of a couplet, **aḥ** is pronounced **aha**, and **iḥ** is pronounced **ihi**.

The guttural consonants—**k, kh, g, gh,** and **ṅ**—are pronounced from the throat in much the same manner as in English. **K** is pronounced as in **k**ite, **kh** as in Ec**kh**art, **g** as in **g**ive, **gh** as in di**g h**ard, and **ṅ** as in si**ng.**

The palatal consonants—**c, ch, j, jh,** and **ṣ**—are pronounced with the tongue touching the Þrm ridge behind the teeth. **C** is pronounced as in **ch**air, **ch** as in staun**ch-h**eart, **j** as in **j**oy, **jh** as in he**dgeh**og, and **ṣ** as in ca**n**yon.

The cerebral consonants—**ṭ, ṭh, ḍ, ḍh,** and **ṇ**—are pronounced with the tip of the tongue turned up and drawn back against the dome of the palate. **Ṭ** is pronounced as in **t**ub, **ṭh** as in ligh**t-h**eart, **ḍ** as in **d**ove, **ḍh** as in re**d-h**ot, and **ṇ** as in **n**ut. The dental consonants**—t, th, d, dh,** and **n—**are pronounced in the same manner as the cerebrals, but with the forepart of the tongue against the teeth.

The labial consonants**—p, ph, b, bh,** and **m**—are pronounced with the lips. **P** is pronounced as in **p**ine, **ph** as in u**ph**ill, **b** as in **b**ird, **bh** as in ru**b-h**ard, and **m** as in **m**other.

The semivowels—**y, r, l,** and **v**—are pronounced as in **y**es, **r**un, **l**ight, and **v**ine respectively. The sibilants—**ś, ṣ,** and **s**—are pronounced, respectively, as in the German word **s***prechen* and the English words **sh**ine and **s**un. The letter **h** is pronounced as in **h**ome.

Glossary

A

Absolute Truth—the ultimate source of all energies.

Adhibhautika misery—misery caused by other living beings.

Adhidaivika misery—misery caused by nature.

Adhyātmika misery—misery caused by one's own body and mind.

Advaita (advaita-vāda)—an atheistic philosophy that says all distinctions are but material illusions. *See also:* Māyāvādīs.

Ahaṅkāra—false ego, by which the soul misidentifies with the material body.

Ajāmila—a fallen *brāhmaṇa* who was saved from hell by chanting the name of Lord Nārāyaṇa at the time of death.

Aṣṭāṅga-yoga—the eight-stage mystic *yoga* system propounded by Patañjali. It consists of *yama* and *niyama* (moral practices), *āsana* (bodily postures), *prāṇāyāma* (breath control), *pratyāhāra* (sensory withdrawal), *dhāraṇā* (steadying the mind), *dhyāna* (meditation), and *samādhi* (deep contemplation on Viṣṇu within the heart).

B

Bhagavad-gītā—the discourse between the Supreme Lord, Kṛṣṇa, and His devotee Arjuna expounding devotional service as both the principal means and the ultimate end of spiritual perfection.

Bhagavān—the Supreme Lord, who possesses all opulences in full.

Bhakti-rasāmṛta-sindhu—Rūpa Gosvāmī's definitive explanation of the science of devotional service. Written in Sanskrit, it has been translated by Śrīla Prabhupāda under the title *The Nectar of Devotion.*

Bhaktivinoda Ṭhākura (1838–1915)—the great-grandfather of the present-day Kṛṣṇa consciousness movement. He was the spiritual master of Śrīla Gaurakiśora dāsa Bābājī and father of Śrīla Bhaktisiddhānta Sarasvatī, who was the spiritual master of Śrīla Prabhupāda.

Bhakti—*See: Bhakti-yoga*

Bhakti-yoga—linking with the Supreme Lord through devotional service.

Bharata Mahārāja—an ancient king of India from whom the Pāṇḍavas descended. A great devotee of the Lord, he developed an attachment to a young deer, causing him to take birth as a deer. In his next life, as the *brāhmaṇa* Jaḍa Bharata, he attained spiritual perfection.

Bhārata-varṣa—India, named after King Bharata.

Brahmā—the first created living being and secondary creator of the material universe.

Brahma-bhūta—the joyful state free of material contamination; liberation.

Brahmacārī—one in the first order of spiritual life; a celibate student of a spiritual master.

Brahman—(1) the individual soul; (2) the impersonal, all-pervasive aspect of the Supreme; (3) the Supreme Personality of Godhead ; (4) the *mahat-tattva,* or total material substance.

Brāhmaṇa—a person wise in Vedic knowledge, fixed in goodness, and knowledgeable of Brahman, the Absolute Truth; a member of the first Vedic social order.

Brahma-saṁhitā—a very ancient Sanskrit scripture recording the prayers of Brahmā to the Supreme Lord, Govinda.

C

Caitanya-caritāmṛta—a biography of Śrī Caitanya Mahāprabhu composed in Bengali in the late sixteenth century by Śrīla Kṛṣṇadāsa Kavirāja. Śrīla Prabhupāda produced an elaborate edition in English with extensive commentary.

Caitanya Mahāprabhu (1486–1534)—the Supreme Lord appearing as His own greatest devotee to teach love of God, especially through the process of congregational chanting of His holy names.

D

Deity of the Lord—the authorized form of Kṛṣṇa worshiped in temples.

Demigod—a universal controller and resident of one of the higher planets.

Dharma—religion; duty, especially everyone's eternal service nature.

Dhyāna-yoga—*See: Aṣṭāṅga-yoga*

Dhruva Mahārāja—a great devotee who as a child performed severe austerities to meet the Lord and get the kingdom denied him. He received an entire planet and God realization as well.

F

False ego—the conception that "I am this material body."

G

Garbhodakaśāyī Viṣṇu—the second Viṣṇu expansion, who enters each universe and from whose navel grows a lotus upon which Lord Brahmā appears. Brahmā then creates the diverse material manifestations.

Gopīs—Kṛṣṇa's cowherd girlfriends, who are His most surrendered and confidential devotees.

Govinda—the Supreme Lord, Kṛṣṇa, who gives pleasure to the land, the senses, and the cows.

Gṛhastha—regulated householder life; the second order of Vedic spiritual life; one in that order.

Guru—a spiritual master.

H

Hare Kṛṣṇa mantra—the great chant for deliverance: Hare Kṛṣṇa, Hare Kṛṣṇa, Kṛṣṇa Kṛṣṇa, Hare Hare/ Hare Rāma, Hare Rāma, Rāma Rāma, Hare Hare.

J

Jīva (jīvātmā)—the living entity, who is an eternal individual soul, part and parcel of the Supreme Lord.

Jīva-tattva—the living entities, atomic parts of the Supreme Lord.

Jñāna-yoga—the path of spiritual realization through a speculative philosophical search for truth.

K

Kali—the presiding personality of Kali-yuga.

Kali, Age of—*See:* Kali-yuga.

Kali-yuga (Age of Kali)—the present age, characterized by quarrel. It is last in the cycle of four ages and began five thousand years ago.

Karma—(1) material action performed according to scriptural regulations; (2) action pertaining to the development of the material body; (3) any material action which will incur a subsequent reaction; (4) the material reaction one incurs due to fruitive activities.

Kṛṣṇa—the original, two-armed form of the Supreme Personality of Godhead.

Kṛṣṇadāsa Kavirāja—the great Vaiṣṇava spiritual master who recorded the biography and teachings of Lord Caitanya Mahāprabhu in his *Caitanya-caritāmṛta*.

Kṣatriya—a warrior or administrator; the second Vedic social order.

Kṣīrodakaśāyī Viṣṇu—the expansion of the Supreme Lord who enters the heart of every living being as the Supersoul.

Kurukṣetra—a place of pilgrimage held sacred since ancient times and the site of a great war fought five thousand years ago; located near New Delhi, India.

Kurus—the descendants of Kuru, especially the sons of Dhṛtarāṣṭra, who were enemies of the Pāṇḍavas.

M

Madhvācārya—a great thirteenth-century Vaiṣṇava spiritual master who preached the theistic philosophy of pure dualism, the duality between the soul and God.

Mahābhārata—Vyāsadeva's epic history of greater India, which includes the events of the Kurukṣetra war and the narration of the *Bhagavad-gītā.*

Mahā-mantra—the great chant for deliverance: Hare Kṛṣṇa, Hare Kṛṣṇa, Kṛṣṇa Kṛṣṇa, Hare Hare/ Hare Rāma, Hare Rāma, Rāma Rāma, Hare Hare.

Mahārāja Parīkṣit—*See:* Parīkṣit Mahārāja

Mahā-Viṣṇu—the expansion of the Supreme Lord from whom all material universes emanate.

Mantra—a transcendental sound or Vedic hymn that can deliver the mind from illusion.

Manu—a demigod son of Brahmā who is the forefather and lawgiver of the human race. There is a succession of fourteen Manus during each day of Brahmā.

Manvantara-avatāras—the special incarnations of the Supreme Lord who appear during the reign of each Manu.

Māyā—the inferior, illusory energy of the Supreme Lord, which rules over this material creation; also, forgetfulness of one's relationship with Kṛṣṇa.

Māyāvādīs—impersonalist philosophers who conceive of the Absolute as ultimately formless and the living entity as equal to God .

Mukti—liberation from material bondage.

Mumbai—the former Bombay.

N

Nārada Muni—a pure devotee of the Lord who travels throughout the universes in his eternal body, glorifying devotional service. He is the spiritual master of Vyāsadeva and of many other great devotees.

Nārada-pañcarātra—Nārada Muni's book on the processes of

Deity worship and *mantra* meditation.

Nārāyaṇa, Lord—the Supreme Lord in His majestic, four-armed form. An expansion of Kṛṣṇa, He presides over the Vaikuṇṭha planets.

Narottama Dāsa Ṭhākura—an exalted devotee of Lord Caitanya who lived in the sixteenth century. He is known especially for his devotional songs written in simple Bengali but containing the highest spiritual truths.

Niyama—*See: Aṣṭāṅga-yoga*

Nṛsiṁhadeva—the half-man, half-lion incarnation of the Supreme Lord, who protected Prahlāda and killed the demon Hiraṇyakaśipu.

P

Pāṇḍavas—Yudhiṣṭhira, Bhīma, Arjuna, Nakula, and Sahadeva, the five warrior-brothers who were intimate friends and devotees of Lord Kṛṣṇa.

Parabrahman—the Supreme Absolute Truth as the Personality of Godhead—Viṣṇu, or Kṛṣṇa.

Paramātmā—the Supersoul, a Viṣṇu expansion of the Supreme Lord residing in the heart of each embodied living entity and pervading all of material nature.

Parīkṣit Mahārāja—the emperor of the world who heard *Śrīmad-Bhāgavatam* from Śukadeva Gosvāmī and thus attained perfection.

Prahlāda Mahārāja—a devotee persecuted by his demoniac father, Hiraṇyakaśipu, but protected and saved by the Lord in the form of Nṛsiṁhadeva.

Prakṛti—the energy of the Supreme; the female principle enjoyed by the male *puruṣa*.

Prasādam—the Lord's mercy; food or other items spiritualized by being first offered to the Supreme Lord.

Puruṣa—the enjoyer, or male; the living entity or the Supreme Lord.

Puruṣa-avatāras—the three primary Viṣṇu expansions of the Supreme Lord who are involved in universal creation. *See* *also:* Garbhodakaśāyī Viṣṇu, Kṣīrodakaśāyī Viṣṇu, Mahā-Viṣṇu

R

Rādhā—*See:* Rādhārāṇī

Rādhārāṇī—Lord Kṛṣṇa's most intimate consort, who is the personification of His internal, spiritual potency.

Rāmānujācārya—a great eleventh-century spiritual master of the Śrī Vaiṣṇava *sampradāya.*

Ṛṣabhadeva—an incarnation of the Supreme Lord as a devotee king who, after instructing his sons in spiritual life, renounced His kingdom for a life of austerity.

Rūpa Gosvāmī—the chief of the six Vaiṣṇava spiritual masters who directly followed Lord Caitanya Mahāprabhu and systematically presented His teachings.

S

Śaktyāveśa-avatāra—a living entity empowered by the Supreme Lord with one or more of His energies or opulences.

Sampradāya—a disciplic succession of spiritual masters; the followers in that tradition.

Sanātana Gosvāmī—one of the six Vaiṣṇava spiritual masters who directly followed Lord Caitanya Mahāprabhu and systematically presented His teachings.

Śaṅkarācārya—the incarnation of Lord Śiva as the great philosopher who, on the order of the Supreme Lord, preached impersonalism based on the *Vedas*.

Sannyāsa—renounced life; the fourth order of Vedic spiritual life.

Sannyāsī—one in the *sannyāsa* (renounced) order.

Śāstra—revealed scripture, such as the Vedic literature.

Śiva—the special incarnation of the Lord as the demigod in charge of the mode of ignorance and the destruction of the material manifestation.

Śrīla—a title indicating possession of exceptional spiritual qualities.

Śrīla Kṛṣṇadāsa Kavirāja Gosvāmī—*See:* Kṛṣṇadāsa Kavirāja

Śrīla Prabhupāda—His Divine Grace A. C. Bhaktivedanta Swami Prabhupāda.

Śrīla Rūpa Gosvāmī—*See:* Rūpa Gosvāmī

Śrīla Sanātana Gosvāmī— *See:* Sanātana Gosvāmī

Śrīmad-Bhāgavatam—the *Purāṇa,* or history, written by Śrīla Vyāsadeva specifically to give a deep understanding of Lord Kṛṣṇa, His devotees, and devotional service.

Śrīmatī Rādhārāṇī—*See:* Rādhārāṇī

Śruti—knowledge via hearing; also, the original Vedic scriptures (the *Vedas* and *Upaniṣads*), given directly by the Supreme Lord.

Śūdra—a laborer; the fourth of the Vedic social orders.

Śukadeva Gosvāmī—the great devotee sage who spoke *Śrīmad-Bhāgavatam* to King Parīkṣit just prior to the king's death.

T

Threefold miseries—*See: Adhibhautika* misery; *Adhidaivika* misery; *Adhyātmika* misery.

U

Upaniṣads—108 philosophical works that appear within the *Vedas*.

V

Vaikuṇṭha—the spiritual world, where there is no anxiety.

Vaiṣṇava—a devotee of Lord Viṣṇu, or Kṛṣṇa.

Vaiśya—a farmer or merchant; the third Vedic social order.

Vānaprastha—one who has retired from family life; the third order of Vedic spiritual life.

Vedānta—the philosophy of the *Vedānta-sūtra* of Śrīla Vyāsadeva. It contains a conclusive summary of Vedic philosophical knowledge and shows Kṛṣṇa to be the goal.

Vedānta-sūtra—the philosophical treatise written by Vyāsadeva, consisting of aphorisms that embody the essential meaning of the *Upaniṣads*.

Vedas—the four original revealed scriptures (*Ṛg, Sāma, Atharva,* and *Yajur*).

Vedic—pertaining to a culture in which all aspects of human life are under the guidance of the *Vedas*.

Viṣṇu Purāṇa—one of the eighteen *Purāṇas,* or Vedic historical scriptures.

Viṣṇu(s)—the Supreme Lord; Lord Kṛṣṇa's expansions in Vaikuṇṭha and for the creation and maintenance of the material universes.

Viṣṇu-tattva—the status or category of Godhead; primary expansions of the Supreme Lord.

Vṛndāvana—Kṛṣṇa's eternal abode, where He fully manifests His quality of sweetness; the village on this earth in which He enacted His childhood pastimes five thousand years ago.

Vyāsadeva—the incarnation of Lord Kṛṣṇa who gave the *Vedas, Purāṇas, Vedānta-sūtra,* and *Mahābhārata* to mankind.

Y

Yama—*See: Aṣṭāṅga-yoga*

Yoga—spiritual discipline undergone to link oneself with the Supreme.

Yogī—a transcendentalist striving for union with the Supreme.

The International Society for Krishna Consciousness
Founder-Acarya: His Divine Grace A.C. Bhaktivedanta Swami Prabhupada

CENTERS AROUND THE WORLD

(September 1997)

NORTH AMERICA

CANADA

Calgary, Alberta — 313 Fourth Street N.E., T2E 3S3/ Tel. (403) 265-3302
Edmonton, Alberta — 9353 35th Avenue, T6E 5R5/ Tel. (403) 439-9999
Montreal, Quebec — 1626 Pie IX Boulevard, H1V 2C5/ Tel. (514) 521-1301
Ottawa, Ontario — 212 Somerset St. E., K1N 6V4/ Tel. (613) 565-6544
Regina, Saskatchewan — 1279 Retallack St., S4T 2H8/ Tel. (306) 525-1640
Toronto, Ontario — 243 Avenue Rd., M5R 2J6/ Tel. (416) 922-5415
Vancouver, B.C. — 5462 S.E. Marine Dr., Burnaby V5J 3G8/ Tel. (604) 433-9728
Victoria, B.C. — 1350 Lang St., V8T 2S5/ Tel. (604) 920-0026

FARM COMMUNITY

Ashcroft, B.C. — Saranagati Dhama, Box 99, V0K 1A0

ADDITIONAL RESTAURANT

Vancouver — Hare Krishna Place, 46 Begbie St., New Westminster

U.S.A.

Atlanta, Georgia — 1287 South Ponce de Leon Ave. N.E., 30306/ Tel. (404) 378-9234
Austin, Texas — 807-A E. 30th St., 78705/ Tel. (512) 320-0477/ E-mail: sankarsana@aol.com
Baltimore, Maryland — 200 Bloomsbury Ave., Catonsville, 21228/ Tel. (410) 744-1624 or 4069
Boise, Idaho — 1615 Martha St., 83706/ Tel. (208) 344-4274
Boston, Massachusetts — 72 Commonwealth Ave., 02116/ Tel. (617) 247-8611
Chicago, Illinois — 1716 W. Lunt Ave., 60626/ Tel. (312) 973-0900
Columbus, Ohio — 379 W. Eighth Ave., 43201/ Tel. (614) 421-1661
Dallas, Texas — 5430 Gurley Ave., 75223/ Tel. (214) 827-6330
Denver, Colorado — 1400 Cherry St., 80220/ Tel. (303) 333-5461
Detroit, Michigan — 383 Lenox Ave., 48215/ Tel. (313) 824-6000
Gainesville, Florida — 214 N.W. 14th St., 32603/ Tel. (904) 336-4183
Gurabo, Puerto Rico — HC01-Box 8440, 00778-9763/ Tel. (809) 737-1658
Hartford, Connecticut — 1683 Main St., E. Hartford, 06108/ Tel. (860) 289-7252
Honolulu, Hawaii — 51 Coelho Way, 96817/ Tel. (808) 595-3947
Houston, Texas — 1320 W. 34th St., 77018/ Tel. (713) 686-4482
Laguna Beach, California — 285 Legion St., 92651/ Tel. (714) 494-7029
Long Island, New York — 197 S. Ocean Avenue, Freeport, 11520/ Tel. (516) 223-4909
Los Angeles, California — 3764 Watseka Ave., 90034/ Tel. (310) 836-2676
Miami, Florida — 3220 Virginia St., 33133 (mail: P.O. Box 337, Coconut Grove, FL 33233)/Tel. (305) 442-7218
New Orleans, Louisiana — 2936 Esplanade Ave., 70119/ Tel. (504) 486-3583
New York, New York — 305 Schermerhorn St., Brooklyn, 11217/ Tel. (718) 855-6714
New York, New York — 26 Second Avenue, 10003/ Tel. (212) 420-1130
Philadelphia, Pennsylvania — 41 West Allens Lane, 19119/ Tel. (215) 247-4600
Phoenix, Arizona — 100 S. Weber Dr., Chandler, 85226/ Tel. (602) 705-4900/ Fax: (602) 705-4901
Portland, Oregon — 5137 N.E. 42 Ave., 97218/ Tel. (503) 287-3252
St. Louis, Missouri — 3926 Lindell Blvd., 63108/ Tel. (314) 535-8085
San Diego, California — 1030 Grand Ave., Pacific Beach, 92109/ Tel. (619) 483-2500
Seattle, Washington — 1420 228th Ave. S.E., Issaquah, 98027/ Tel. (206) 391-3293
Tallahassee, Florida — 1323 Nylic St. (mail: P.O. Box 20224, 32304)/ Tel. (904) 681-9258
Towaco, New Jersey — P.O. Box 109, 07082/ Tel. (201) 299-0970
Tucson, Arizona — 711 E. Blacklidge Dr., 85719/ Tel. (520) 792-0630
Washington, D.C. — 3200 Ivy Way, Harwood, MD 20776/ Tel. (301) 261-4493
Washington, D.C. — 10310 Oaklyn Dr., Potomac, Maryland 20854/ Tel. (301) 299-2100

FARM COMMUNITIES

Alachua, Florida (New Raman Reti) — P.O. Box 819, 32615/ Tel. (904) 462-2017
Carriere, Mississippi (New Talavan) — 31492 Anner Road, 39426/ Tel. (601) 799-1354
Gurabo, Puerto Rico (New Govardhana Hill) — (contact ISKCON Gurabo)
Hillsborough, North Carolina (New Goloka) — 1032 Dimmocks Mill Rd., 27278/ Tel. (919) 732-6492
Moundsville, West Virginia (New Vrindaban) — R.D. No. 1, Box 319, Hare Krishna Ridge, 26042/ Tel. (304) 843-1600/ Fax: (304) 845-9819/ E-mail: story 108@juno.com; (lodging:) kisore@aol.com
Mulberry, Tennessee (Murari-sevaka) — Rt. No. 1, Box 146-A, 37359/ Tel (615) 759-6888
Port Royal, Pennsylvania (Gita Nagari) — R.D. No. 1, Box 839, 17082/ Tel. (717) 527-4101

ADDITIONAL RESTAURANTS AND DINING

Boise, Idaho — Govinda's, 500 W. Main St., 83702/ Tel. (208) 338-9710
Eugene, Oregon — Govinda's Vegetarian Buffet, 270 W. 8th St., 97401/ Tel. (503) 686-3531
Fresno, California — Govinda's, 2373 E. Shaw, 93710/ Tel. (209) 225-1230
Gainesville, Florida — Radha's, 125 NW 23rd Ave., 32609/ Tel. (904) 376-9012

EUROPE

UNITED KINGDOM AND IRELAND

Belfast, Northern Ireland — 140 Upper Dunmurray Lane, BT17 OHE/ Tel. +44 (01232) 620530

Birmingham, England — 84 Stanmore Rd., Edgebaston, B16 9TB/ Tel. +44 (0121) 420-4999
Coventry, England — Sri Sri Radha Krishna Cultural Centre, Kingfield Rd., Radford (mail: 19 Gloucester St., CV1 3BZ)/ Tel. +44 (01203) 555420
Dublin, Ireland — 56 Dame St., Dublin 2/ Tel. +353 (01) 679-1306
Glasgow, Scotland — Karuna Bhavan, Bankhouse Rd., Lesmahagow, Lanarkshire ML11 0ES/Tel. +44 (01555) 894790
Leicester, England — 21 Thoresby St., North Evington, Leicester LE5 4GU/Tel. +44 (0116) 2762587 or 2367723
Liverpool, England — 114A Bold St., Liverpool L1 4HY/ Tel. +44 (0151) 708 9400
London, England (city) — 10 Soho St., London W1V 5DA/ Tel. +44 (0171) 4373662 (business hours), 4393606 (other times); Govinda's Restaurant: 4374928
London, England (country) — Bhaktivedanta Manor, Letchmore Heath, Watford, Hertfordshire WD2 8EP/ Tel. +44 (01923) 857244
London, England (south) — 42 Enmore Road, South Norwood, London SE25/ Tel. +44 (0181) 656-4296
Manchester, England — 20 Mayfield Rd., Whalley Range, Manchester M16 8FT/ Tel. +44 (0161) 2264416
Newcastle upon Tyne, England — 21 Leazes Park Rd., NE1 4PF/ Tel. +44 (0191) 2220150

FARM COMMUNITIES
County Wicklow, Ireland — Rathgorragh, Kiltegan/ Tel. +353 508-73305
Lisnaskea, North Ireland — Hare Krishna Island, BT92 9GN Lisnaskea, Co. Fremanagh/Tel. +44 (03657) 21512
London, England — (contact Bhaktivedanta Manor)

ADDITIONAL RESTAURANT
Manchester, England — Krishna's, 20 Cyril St., Manchester 14/ Tel. +44 (0161) 226 965
(Krishna conscious programs are held regularly in more than twenty other cities in the U.K. For information, contact Bhaktivedanta Books Ltd., Reader Services Dept., P.O. Box 324, Borehamwood, Herts WD6 1NB/ Tel. +44 [0181] 905-1244.)

GERMANY
Abentheuer — Bockingstr 8, 55767 Abentheuer/ Tel. +49 (06782) 6364
Berlin — Johannisthaler Chaussee 78, 12259 Berlin (Britz)/ Tel. +49 (030) 613 2400
Boeblingen — Friedrich-List Strasse 58, 71032 Boeblingen/ Tel. +49 (07031) 22 33 98
Cologne — Taunusstr. 40, 51105 Köln/ Tel. +49 (0221) 830 3778
Flensburg— Hoerup 1, 24980 Neuhoerup/ Tel. +49 (04639) 73 36
Hamburg — Muehlenstr. 93, 25421 Pinneberg/ Tel. +49 (04101) 2 39 31
Hannover — Zeiss Strasse 21, 30519 Hannover/ Tel. +49 (0511) 83 74 31
Heidelberg — Kurfürsten-Anlage 5, D-69115 Heidelberg/ Tel. +49 (06221) 16 51 01
Munich — Tal 38, 80331 Munchen/ Tel +49 (089) 29 23 17
Nuremberg — Kopernikusplatz 12, 90459 Nürnberg/ Tel. +49 (0911) 45 32 86
Wiesbaden — Schiersteiner Strasse 6, 65187 Wiesbaden/ Tel. +49 (0611) 37 33 12

FARM COMMUNITY
Jandelsbrunn — Nava Jiyada Nrsimha Ksetra, Zielberg 20, 94118 Jandelsbrunn/ Tel +49 (08583) 316

ADDITIONAL RESTAURANT
Berlin — Higher Taste, Kurfuerstendamm 157/158, 10709 Berlin/ Tel. +49 (030) 892 99 17

ITALY
Asti — Roatto, Frazione Valle Reale 20/ Tel. +39 (0141) 938406
Bergamo — Villaggio Hare Krishna, Via Galileo Galilei 41, 24040 Chignolo D'isola (BG)/Tel. +39 (035) 4940706
Bologna — Via Ramo Barchetta 2, 40010 Bentivoglio (BO)/ Tel. +39 (051) 863924
Catania — Via San Nicolo al Borgo 28, 95128 Catania, Sicily/ Tel. +39 (095) 522-252
Naples — Via Vesuvio, N33, Ercolano LNA7/ Tel. +39 (081) 739-0398
Rome — Nepi, Sri Gaura Mandala, Via Mazzanese Km. 0,700 (dalla Cassia uscita Calcata), Pian del Pavone (Viterbo)/ Tel. +39 (0761) 527038
Vicenza — Via Roma 9, 36020 Albettone (Vicenza)/ Tel. +39 (0444) 790573 or 790566

FARM COMMUNITY
Florence (Villa Vrindavan) — Via Communale degli Scopeti 108, S. Andrea in Percussina, San Casciano, Val di Pesa (FI) 5002/ Tel. +39 (055) 820-054

ADDITIONAL RESTAURANT
Milan — Govinda's, Via Valpetrosa 3/5, 20123 Milano/ Tel. +39 (02) 862-417

POLAND
Augustow — ul Arnikowa 5, 16-300 Augustow/ Tel. & fax +48 (119) 46147
Bedzin — ul. Promyka 31, 42-500 Bedzin
Gdansk — ul. Cedrowa 5, Gdansk 80-125 (mail: MTSK 80-958 Gdansk 50 skr. poczt. 364)/ Tel. +48 (58) 329665
Krakow — ul. Podedworze 23a, 30-686 Krakow/ Tel. +48 (12) 588283
Lublin — ul Bursztynowa 12/52 (mail: Hare Kryszna, 20-001 Lublin 1, P.O. Box 196)/ Tel. +48 (81) 560685
Walbrzych — ul Schmidta 1/5, 58-300 Walbrzych/ Tel. +48 (74) 23185
Warsaw — Mysiadlo k. Warszawy, ul. Zakret 11, 05-500 Piaseczno (mail: MTSK 02-770 Warszawa 130, P.O. Box 257) / Tel. & fax +48 (22) 756-27-11
Wroclaw — ul. Bierutowska 23, 51-317 Wroclaw (mail: MTSK 50-900 Wroclaw, P.O. Box 858)/ Tel. & fax +48 (71) 250-981

FARM COMMUNITY
New Santipura — Czarnow 21, k. Kamiennej gory, woj. Jelenia gora/ Tel. +48 8745-1892

SWEDEN
Gothenburg — Hojdgatan 22, 431 36 Moelndal/ Tel. +46 (031) 879648
Grödinge — Korsnäs Gård, 14792 Grödinge/ Tel. +46 (8530) 29151

Karlstad — Vastra torgg. 16, 65224 Karlstad
Lund — Bredgatan 28 ipg, 222 21/ Tel. +46 (046) 120413
Malmö — Föreningsgatan 28, 21152 Malmö/ Tel. +46 (040) 6116497; restaurant: 6116496
Stockholm — Fridhemsgatan 22, 11240 Stockholm/ Tel. +46 (08) 6549 002
Uppsala — Nannaskolan sal F 3, Kungsgatan 22 (mail: Box 833, 751 08, Uppsala)/ Tel. +46 (018) 102924 or 509956

FARM COMMUNITY
Järna — Almviks Gård, 153 95 Järna/ Tel. +46 (8551) 52050; 52105

ADDITIONAL RESTAURANTS
Göthenburg — Govinda's, Storgatan 20,S-411 38 Göthenburg / Tel. +46 (031) 139698
Malmö — Higher Taste, Amiralsgatan 6, S-211 55 Malmö/ Tel. +46 (040) 970600
Umea — Govinda's, Pilg. 28, 90331 Umea/ Tel. +46 (090) 178875

SWITZERLAND

Basel — Hammerstrasse 11, 4058 Basel/ Tel. +41 (061) 693 26 38
Bern — Marktgasse 7, 3011 Bern/ Tel. +41 (031) 312 38 25
Lugano — Via ai Grotti, 6862 Rancate (TI)/ Tel. +41 (091) 646 66 16
Zürich — Bergstrasse 54, 8030 Zürich/ Tel. +41 (1) 262-33-88
Zürich — Preyergrasse 16, 8001 Zürich/ Tel. +41 (1) 251-88-59

OTHER COUNTRIES

Amsterdam, The Netherlands — Van Hilligaertstraat 17, 1072 JX, Amsterdam/ Tel. +31 (020) 6751404
Antwerp, Belgium — Amerikalei 184, 2000 Antwerpen/ Tel. +32 (03) 237-0037
Barcelona, Spain — c/de L'Oblit 67, 08026 Barcelona/ Tel. +34 (93) 347-9933
Belgrade, Serbia — VVZ-Veda, Custendilska 17, 11000 Beograd/ Tel. +381 (11) 781-695
Budapest, Hungary — Hare Krishna Temple, Mariaremetei ut. 77, Budapest 1028 II/Tel. +36 (01) 1768774
Copenhagen, Denmark — Baunevej 23, 3400 Hillerød/ Tel. +45 42286446
Debrecen, Hungary — L. Hegyi Mihalyne, U62, Debrecen 4030/ Tel. +36 (052) 342-496
Helsinki, Finland — Ruoholahdenkatu 24 D (III krs) 00180, Helsinki/ Tel. +358 (0) 6949879
Iasi, Romania — Stradela Moara De Vint 72, 6600 Iasi
Kaunas, Lithuania — Savanoryu 37, Kaunas/ Tel. +370 (07) 222574
Ljubljana, Slovenia — Zibertova 27, 61000 Ljubljana/ Tel. +386 (061) 131-23-19
Madrid, Spain — Espíritu Santo 19, 28004 Madrid/ Tel. +34 (91) 521-3096
Málaga, Spain — Ctra. Alora, 3 int., 29140 Churriana/ Tel. +34 (952) 621038
Oslo, Norway — Jonsrudvej 1G, 0274 Oslo/ Tel. +47 (022) 552243
Paris, France — 31 Rue Jean Vacquier, 93160 Noisy le Grand/ Tel. +33 (01) 43043263
Plovdiv, Bulgaria — ul. Prosveta 56, Kv. Proslav, Plovdiv 4015/ Tel. +359 (032) 446962
Porto, Portugal — Rua S. Miguel, 19 C.P. 4000 (mail: Apartado 4108, 4002 Porto Codex)/ Tel. +351 (02) 2005469
Prague, Czech Republic — Jilova 290, Prague 5-Zlicin 155 00/ Tel. +42 (02) 3021282 or 3021608
Pula, Croatia — Vinkuran centar 58, 52000 Pula (mail: P.O. Box 16)/ Tel. & fax +385 (052) 573581
Rijeka, Croatia — Svetog Jurja 32, 51000 Rijeka (mail: P.O. Box 61)/ Tel. & fax +385 (051) 263404
Riga, Latvia — 56 Krishyana Barona, LV 1011/ Tel. +371 (02) 272490
Rotterdam, The Netherlands — Braamberg 45, 2905 BK Capelle a/d Yssel./ Tel. +31 (010) 4580873
Santa Cruz de Tenerife, Spain — C/ Castillo, 44, 4°, Santa Cruz 38003,Tenerife/ Tel. +34 (922) 241035
Sarajevo, Bosnia-Herzegovina — Saburina 11, 71000 Sarajevo/ Tel. +381 (071) 531-154
Septon-Durbuy, Belgium — Chateau de Petite Somme, 6940 Septon-Durbuy/ Tel. +32 (086) 322926
Skopje, Macedonia — Vvz. "ISKCON," Roze Luksemburg 13, 91000 Skopje/ Tel. +389 (091) 201451
Sofia, Bulgaria — Villa 3, Vilna Zona-Iztok, Simeonovo, Sofia 1434/ Tel. +359 (02) 6352608
Split, Croatia — Cesta Mutogras 26, 21312 Podstrana, Split (mail: P.O. Box 290, 21001 Split)/ Tel. +385 (021) 651137
Tallinn, Estonia — ul Linnamae Tee 11-97/ Tel. +372 (0142) 59756
Timisoara, Romania — ISKCON, Porumbescu 92, 1900 Timisoara/ Tel. +40 (961) 54776
Vienna, Austria — ISKCON, Rosenackerstrasse 26, 1170 Vienna/ Tel. +43 (01) 455830
Vilnius, Lithuania — Raugyklos G. 23-1, 2024 Vilnius/ Tel. +370 (0122) 66-12-18
Zagreb, Croatia — Bizek 5,10000 Zagreb (mail: P.O. Box 68, 10001 Zagreb)/ Tel. & fax +385 (01) 190548

FARM COMMUNITIES
Czech Republic — Krsnuv Dvur c. 1, 257 28 Chotysany
France (Bhaktivedanta Village) — Chateau Bellevue, F-39700 Chatenois/ Tel. +33 (084) 728235
France (La Nouvelle Mayapura) — Domaine d'Oublaisse, 36360, Lucay le Mâle/ Tel. +33 (054) 402481
Spain (New Vraja Mandala) — (Santa Clara) Brihuega, Guadalajara/ Tel. +34 (911) 280018

ADDITIONAL RESTAURANTS
Barcelona, Spain — Restaurante Govinda, Plaza de la Villa de Madrid 4-5, 08002 Barcelona
Copenhagen, Denmark — Govinda's, Noerre Farimagsgade 82/ Tel. +45 33337444
Oslo, Norway — Krishna's Cuisine, Kirkeveien 59B, 0364 Oslo/ Tel. +47 22606250
Prague, Czech Republic — Govinda's, Soukenicka 27, 110 00 Prague-1/ Tel. +42 (02) 2481-6631, 2481-6016
Prague, Czech Republic — Govinda's, Na hrazi 5, 180 00 Prague 8-Liben/ Tel. +42 (02) 683-7226
Vienna, Austria — Govinda, Lindengasse 2A, 1070 Vienna/ Tel. +43 (01) 5222817

C. I. S. (Commonwealth of Independent States)

RUSSIA

Moscow — Khoroshevskoye shosse d.8, korp.3, 125 284, Moscow/ Tel. +7 (095) 255-67-11

Moscow — Nekrasovsky pos., Dmitrovsky reg., 141760 Moscow/ Tel. +7 (095) 979-8268
Nijni Novgorod — ul. Ivana Mochalova, 7-69, 603904 Nijni Novgorod/ Tel. +7 (8312) 252592
Novosibirsk — ul. Leningradskaya 111-20, Novosibirsk
Perm (Ural Region) — Pr. Mira, 113-142, 614065 Perm/ Tel. +7 (3442) 335740
St. Petersburg — 17, Bumazhnaya st., 198020 St. Petersburg/ Tel. +7 (0812) 186-7259
Ulyanovsk — ul Glinki, 10 /Tel. +7 (0842) 221-42-89
Vladivostok — ul. Ridneva 5-1, 690087 Vladivostok/ Tel. +7 (4232) 268943

UKRAINE

Dnepropetrovsk — ul. Ispolkomovskaya, 56A, 320029 Dnepropetrovsk/ Tel. +380 (0562) 445029
Donetsk — ul. Tubensa, 22, 339018 Makeyevka/ Tel. +380 (0622) 949104
Kharkov — ul. Verhnyogievskaya, 43, 310015 Kharkov/ Tel. +380 (0572) 202167 or 726968
Kiev — ul. Menjinskogo, 21-B., 252054 Kiev/Tel. +380 (044) 2444944
Nikolayev — Sudostroitelny pereulok, 5/8, Nikolayev 327052/ Tel. +380 (0512) 351734
Simferopol — ul. Kievskaya 149/15, 333000 Simferopol/ Tel. +380 (0652) 225116
Vinnitza — ul. Chkalov St., 5, Vinnitza 26800/ Tel. +380 (0432) 323152

OTHER COUNTRIES

Alma Ata, Kazakstan — Per Kommunarov, 5, 480022 Alma Ata/ Tel. +7 (3272) 353830
Baku, Azerbaijan — Pos. 8-i km, per. Sardobi 2, Baku 370060/ Tel. +7 (8922) 212376
Bishkek, Kyrgizstan — Per. Omski, 5, 720000 Bishkek/ Tel. +7 (3312) 472683
Dushanbe, Tadjikistan — ul Anzob, 38, 724001 Dushanbe/ Tel. +7 (3772) 271830
Kishinev, Moldova — ul. Popovich 13, Kishinev/ Tel. +7 (0422) 558099
Minsk, Belarus — ul. Pavlova 11, 220 053 Minsk/ Tel. +7 (0172) 37-4751
Sukhumi, Georgia — Pr. Mira 274, Sukhumi
Tbilisi, Georgia — ul. Kacharava, 16, 380044 Tbilisi/ Tel. +7 (8832) 623326
Yerevan, Armenia — ul. Krupskoy 18, 375019 Yerevan/ Tel. +7 (8852) 275106

AUSTRALASIA

AUSTRALIA

Canberra — 15 Parkhill St., Pearce ACT 2607 (mail: GPO Box 1411, Canberra 2601)/ Tel. +61 (06) 290-1869
Melbourne — 197 Danks St., Albert Park, Victoria 3206 (mail: P.O. Box 125)/ Tel. +61 (03) 969 95122
Perth — 356 Murray St., Perth (mail: P.O. Box 102, Bayswater, W. A. 6053)/ Tel. +61 (09) 481-1114 or 370-1552 (evenings)
Sydney — 180 Falcon St., North Sydney, N.S.W. 2060 (mail: P. O. Box 459, Cammeray, N.S.W.2062)/ Tel. +61 (02) 9959-4558
Sydney — 3296 King St., Newtown 2042/ Tel. +61 (02) 550-6524

FARM COMMUNITIES

Bambra (New Nandagram) — Oak Hill, Dean's Marsh Rd., Bambra, VIC 3241/ Tel. +61 (052) 88-7383
Millfield, N.S.W. — New Gokula Farm, Lewis Lane (off Mt.View Rd. Millfield near Cessnock), N.S.W. (mail: P.O. Box 399, Cessnock 2325, N.S.W.)/ Tel. +61 (049) 98-1800
Murwillumbah (New Govardhana) — Tyalgum Rd., Eungella, via Murwillumbah N. S. W. 2484 (mail: P.O. Box 687)/ Tel. +61 (066) 72-6579

ADDITIONAL RESTAURANTS

Adelaide — Food for Life, 79 Hindley St./ Tel. +61 (08) 2315258
Brisbane — Govinda's, 1st •oor, 99 Elizabeth Street/ Tel. +61 (07) 210-0255
Brisbane — Hare Krishna Food for Life, 190 Brunswick St. Fortitude Valley/ Tel. +61 (070) 854-1016
Melbourne — Crossways, Floor 1, 123 Swanston St., Melbourne, Victoria 3000/ Tel. +61 (03) 9650-2939
Melbourne — Gopal's, 139 Swanston St., Melbourne, Victoria 3000/ Tel. +61 (03) 9650-1578
Perth — Hare Krishna Food for Life, 200 William St., Northbridge, WA 6003/ Tel. +61 (09) 227-1684

NEW ZEALAND, FIJI, AND PAPUA NEW GUINEA

Christchurch, New Zealand — 83 Bealey Ave. (mail: P.O. Box 25-190 Christchurch)/ Tel. +64 (03) 3665-174
Labasa, Fiji — Delailabasa (mail: P.O. Box 133)/ Tel. +679 812912
Lautoka, Fiji — 5 Tavewa Ave. (mail: P.O. Box 125)/ Tel. +679 664112
Port Moresby, Papua New Guinea — Section 23, Lot 46, Gordonia St., Hohola (mail: P. O. Box 571, POM NCD)/ Tel. +675 259213
Rakiraki, Fiji — Rewasa, Rakiraki (mail: P.O. Box 204)/ Tel. +679 694243
Suva, Fiji — Nasinu 7½ miles (mail: P.O. Box 7315)/ Tel. +679 393599
Wellington, New Zealand — 60 Wade St., Wadestown, Wellington (mail: P.O. Box 2753, Wellington)/ Tel. +64 (04) 4720510

FARM COMMUNITY

Auckland, New Zealand (New Varshan) — Hwy. 18, Riverhead, next to Huapai Golf Course (mail: R.D. 2, Kumeu, Auckland)/ Tel. +64 (09) 4128075

RESTAURANTS

Auckland, New Zealand — Gopal's, Civic House (1st •oor), 291 Queen St./ Tel. +64 (09) 3034885
Christchurch, New Zealand — Gopal's, 143 Worcester St./ Tel. +64 (03) 3667-035
Labasa, Fiji — Hare Krishna Restaurant, Naseakula Road/ Tel. +679 811364
Lautoka, Fiji — Gopal's, Corner of Yasawa St. and Naviti St./ Tel. +679 662990
Suva, Fiji — Gopal's, 18 Pratt St./ Tel. +679 314154

AFRICA

NIGERIA

Abeokuta — Ibadan Rd., Obanatoka (mail: P.O. Box 5177)

Benin City — 108 Lagos Rd., Uselu/ Tel. +234 (052) 247900
Enugu — 8 Church Close, off College Rd., Housing Estate, Abakpa-Nike
Ibadan — 1 Ayo Akintoba St., Agbowo, University of Ibadan
Jos — 5A Liberty Dam Close, P.O. Box 6557, Jos
Kaduna — 8B Dabo Rd., Kaduna South, P.O. Box 1121, Kaduna
Lagos — 25 Jaiyeola Ajata St., Ajao Estate, off International Airport Express Rd., Lagos (mail: P.O. Box 8793)/ Tel. & Fax +234 (01) 876169
Port Harcourt — Second Tarred Road, Ogwaja Waterside (mail: P.O. Box 4429, Trans Amadi)
Warri — Okwodiete Village, Kilo 8, Effurun/Orerokpe Rd. (mail: P.O. Box 1922, Warri)

SOUTH AFRICA

Cape Town — 17 St. Andrews Rd., Rondebosch 7700/ Tel. +27 (021) 689-1529
Durban — Chatsworth Centre, Chatsworth 4030 (mail: P.O. Box 56003)/ Tel. +27 (31) 433-328
Johannesburg — 14 Goldreich St., Hillbrow 2001 (mail: P.O. Box 10667, Johannesburg 2000)/ Tel. +27 (011) 484-3273
Port Elizabeth — 18 Strand Fontein Rd., 6001 Port Elizabeth/ Tel. & Fax +27 (41) 53 43 30

OTHER COUNTRIES

Gaborone, Botswana — P.O. Box 201003/ Tel. +267 307 768
Kampala, Uganda — Bombo Rd., near Makerere University (mail: P.O. Box 1647, Kampala)
Kisumu, Kenya — P.O. Box 547/ Tel. +254 (035) 42546
Marondera, Zimbabwe — 6 Pine Street (mail: P.O. Box 339)/ Tel. +263 (028) 8877801
Mombasa, Kenya — Hare Krishna House, Sauti Ya Kenya and Kisumu Rds. (mail: P.O. Box 82224, Mombasa)/ Tel. +254 (011) 312248
Nairobi, Kenya — Muhuroni Close, off West Nagara Rd. (mail: P.O. Box 28946, Nairobi)/ Tel. +254 (02) 744365
Phoenix, Mauritius — Hare Krishna Land, Pont Fer, Phoenix (mail: P. O. Box 108, Quartre Bornes, Mauritius)/ Tel. +230 696-5804
Rose Hill, Mauritius — 13 Gordon St./ Tel. +230 454-5275

FARM COMMUNITY

Mauritius (ISKCON Vedic Farm) — Hare Krishna Rd., Vrindaban, Bon Acceuil/ Tel. +230 418-3955

ASIA

INDIA

Agartala, Tripura — Assam-Agartala Rd., Banamalipur, 799001
Ahmedabad, Gujarat — Sattelite Rd., Gandhinagar Highway Crossing, Ahmedabad 380054/ Tel. (079) 6749827, 6749945
Allahabad, U. P. — 161, Kashi Nagar, Baluaghat, Allahabad 211003/ Tel. 653318
Bamanbore, Gujarat — N.H. 8A, Surendra-nagar District
Bangalore, Karnataka — Hare Krishna Hill, 1 'R' Block, Chord Road, Rajaji Nagar 560010/ Tel. (080) 332 1956
Baroda, Gujarat — Hare Krishna Land, Gotri Rd., 390021/ Tel. (0265) 326299 or 331012
Belgaum, Karnataka — Shukravar Peth, Tilak Wadi, 590006
Bhubaneswar, Orissa — National Highway No. 5, Nayapali, 751001/ Tel. (0674) 413517 or 413475
Bombay — (see Mumbai)
Calcutta, W. Bengal — 3C Albert Rd., 700017/ Tel. (033) 2473757 or 2476075
Chandigarh — Hare Krishna Land, Dakshin Marg, Sector 36-B, 160036/ Tel. (0172) 601590 and 603232
Coimbatore, Tamil Nadu — 387, VGR Puram, Dr. Alagesan Rd., 641011/ Tel. (0422) 445978 or 442749
Gangapur, Gujarat — Bhaktivedanta Rajavidyalaya, Krishnalok, Surat-Bardoli Rd. Gangapur, P.O. Gangadhara, Dist. Surat, 394310/Tel. (02,61) 667075
Gauhati, Assam — Ulubari Charali, Gauhati 781001/ Tel. (0361) 31208
Guntur, A.P. — Opp. Sivalayam, Peda Kakani 522509
Hanumkonda, A.P. — Neeladri Rd., Kapuwada, 506011/ Tel. 08712-77399
Haridwar, U.P. — ISKCON, P.O. Box 4, Haridwar, U.P. 249401/ Tel. (0133) 422655
Hyderabad, A.P. — Hare Krishna Land, Nampally Station Rd., 500001/ Tel. (040) 592018 or 552924
Imphal, Manipur — Hare Krishna Land, Airport Road, 795001/ Tel. (0385) 221587
Jaipur, Rajasthan — P.O. Box 270, Jaipur 302001/ Tel. (0141) 364022
Katra, Jammu, and Kashmir — Srila Prabhupada Ashram, Srila Prabhupada Marg, Kalka Mata Mandir, Katra (Vashnov Mata) 182101/ Tel. (01991) 3047
Kurukshetra, Haryana — 369 Gudri Muhalla, Main Bazaar, 132118/ Tel. (1744) 32806 or 33529
Lucknow, Uttar Pradesh — 1 Ashak Nagar, Guru Govind Singh Marg, 226018
Madras, Tamil Nadu — 59, Burkit Rd., T. Nagar, 600017/ Tel. 443266
Mayapur, W. Bengal — Shree Mayapur Chandrodaya Mandir, Shree Mayapur Dham, Dist. Nadia (mail: P.O. Box 10279, Ballyganj, Calcutta 700019)/ Tel. (03472) 45239 or 45240 or 45233
Moirang, Manipur — Nongban Ingkhon, Tidim Rd./ Tel. 795133
Mumbai, Maharashtra (Bombay) — Hare Krishna Land, Juhu 400 049/ Tel. (022) 6206860
Mumbai, Maharashtra — 7 K. M. Munshi Marg, Chowpatty, 400007/ Tel. (022) 3634078
Mumbai, Maharashtra — Shivaji Chowk, Station Rd., Bhayandar (West), Thane 401101/ Tel. (022) 8191920
Nagpur, Maharashtra — 70 Hill Road, Ramnagar, 440010/ Tel. (0712) 529932
New Delhi — Sant Nagar Main Road (Garhi), behind Nehru Place Complex (mail: P. O. Box 7061), 110065/ Tel. (011) 6419701 or 6412058
New Delhi — 14/63, Punjabi Bagh, 110026/ Tel. (011) 5410782
Pandharpur, Maharashtra — Hare Krsna Ashram (across Chandrabhaga River), Dist. Sholapur, 413304/ Tel. (0218) 623473
Patna, Bihar — Rajendra Nagar Road No. 12, 800016/ Tel. (0612) 50765
Pune, Maharashtra — 4 Tarapoor Rd., Camp, 411001/ Tel. (0212) 667259

Puri, Orissa — Sipasurubuli Puri, Dist. Puri/ (06752) 24592, 24594
Puri, Orissa — Bhakti Kuthi, Swargadwar, Puri/ Tel. (06752) 23740
Secunderabad, A.P. — 27 St. John's Road, 500026/ Tel. (040) 805232
Silchar, Assam — Ambikapatti, Silchar, Cachar Dist., 788004
Siliguri, W. Bengal — Gitalpara, 734401/ Tel. (0353) 26619
Surat, Gujarat — Rander Rd., Jahangirpura, 395005/ Tel. (0261) 685516 or 685891
Sri Rangam, Tamal Nadu — 6A E.V.S. Rd., Sri Rangam, Tiruchirapalli 6/ Tel. 433945
Tirupati, A. P. — K.T. Road, Vinayaka Nagar, 517507/ Tel. (08574) 20114
Trivandrum, Kerala — T.C. 224/1485, WC Hospital Rd., Thycaud, 695014/ Tel. (0471) 68197
Udhampur, Jammu and Kashmir — Srila Prabhupada Ashram, Prabhupada Marg, Prabhupada Nagar, Udhampur 182101/ Tel. (01992) 70298
Vallabh Vidyanagar, Gujarat — ISKCON Hare Krishna Land, 338120/ Tel. (02692) 30796
Vrindavana, U. P. — Krishna-Balaram Mandir, Bhaktivedanta Swami Marg, Raman Reti, Mathura Dist., 281124/ Tel. (0565) 442-478 or 442-355

FARM COMMUNITIES

Ahmedabad District, Gujarat — Hare Krishna Farm, Katwada (contact ISKCON Ahmedabad)
Assam — Karnamadhu, Dist. Karimganj
Chamorshi, Maharashtra — 78 Krishnanagar Dham, Dis. Gadhachiroli, 442603

OTHER COUNTRIES

Cagayan de Oro, Philippines — 30 Dahlia St., Ilaya Carmen, 900 (c/o Sepulveda's Compound)
Chittagong, Bangladesh — Caitanya Cultural Society, Sri Pundarik Dham, Mekhala, Hathzari (mail: GPO Box 877, Chittagong)/ Tel. +88 (031) 225822
Colombo, Sri Lanka — 188 New Chetty St., Colombo 13/ Tel. +94 (01) 433325
Dhaka, Bangladesh — 5 Chandra Mohon Basak St., Banagram, Dhaka 1203/ Tel. +880 (02) 236249
Hong Kong — 27 Chatam Road South, 6/F, Kowloon/ Tel. +852 7396818
Iloilo City, Philippines — 13-1-1 Tereos St., La Paz, Iloilo City, Iloilo/ Tel. +63 (033) 73391
Jakarta, Indonesia — P.O. Box 2694, Jakarta Pusat 10001/ Tel. +62 (021) 4899646
Jessore, Bangladesh — Nitai Gaur Mandir, Kathakhali Bazaar, P. O. Panjia, Dist. Jessore
Jessore, Bangladesh — Rupa-Sanatana Smriti Tirtha, Ramsara, P. O. Magura Hat, Dist. Jessore
Kathmandu, Nepal — Budhanilkantha, Kathmandu (mail: P. O. Box 3520)/ Tel. +977 (01) 290743
Kuala Lumpur, Malaysia — Lot 9901, Jalan Awan Jawa, Taman Yarl, off 5½ Mile, Jalan Kelang Lama, Petaling/ Tel. +60 (03) 780-7355, -7360, or -7369
Manila, Philippines — Penthouse Liwag Bldg., 3307 Mantanzas St., Makati, Metro Manila/ Tel. +63 (02) 8337883 loc. 10
Taipei, Taiwan — (mail: c/o ISKCON Hong Kong)
Tel Aviv, Israel — 16 King George St. (mail: P. O. Box 48163, Tel Aviv 61480)/ Tel. +972 (03) 5285475 or 6299011
Tokyo, Japan — 1-29-2-202 Izumi, Suginami-ku, Tokyo 168/ Tel. +81 (03) 3327-1541
Yogyakarta, Indonesia — P.O. Box 25, Babarsari YK, DIY

FARM COMMUNITIES

Indonesia — Govinda Kunja (contact ISKCON Jakarta)
Malaysia — Jalan Sungai Manik, 36000 Teluk Intan, Perak
Philippines (Hare Krishna Paradise) — 231 Pagsabungan Rd., Basak, Mandaue City/ Tel. +63 (032) 83254

ADDITIONAL RESTAURANTS

Cebu, Philippines — Govinda's, 26 Sanchiangko St.
Kuala Lumpur, Malaysia — Govinda's, 16-1 Jalan Bunus Enam, Masjid India/ Tel. +60 (03) 7807355 or 7807360 or 7807369

LATIN AMERICA

BRAZIL

Belém, PA — Almirante Barroso, Travessa Santa Matilde, 64, Souza/ Tel. +55 (091) 243-0558
Belo Horizonte, MG — Rua Aristoteles Caldeira, 334, Prado/ Tel. +55 (031) 332-8460
Brasilia, DF — CLN 310, Bloco B, Loja 45, Terreo/ Tel. +55 (061) 272-3111
Campos, RJ — Rua Barao de Miracema, 186, Centro
Caruaru, PE — Rua Major Sinval, 180, 1º Andar
Curitiba, PR — Al. Cabral, 670, Centro/ Tel. +55 (041) 277-3176
Florianopolis, SC — Rua Laurindo Januario Silveira, 3250, Canto da Lagoa
Fortaleza, CE — Rua Jose Lourenço, 2114, Aldeota/ Tel. +55 (085) 264-1273
Goiania, GO — Rua 24A, 20 (esq. Av. Parananba)/ Tel. +55 (062) 224-9820
Guarulhos, SP — Rua Orixas, 1, Jardim Afonso/ Tel. +55 (011) 209-6669
Manaus, AM — Av. 7 de Setembro, 1599, Centro/ Tel. +55 (092) 232-0202
Petropolis, RJ — Rua do Imperador, 349, Sobrado
Porto Alegre, RS — Av. Basian, 396, Menino Deus/ Tel. +55 (051) 233-1474
Recife, PE — Rua Democlitos de Souza Filho, 235, Madalena
Ribeirao Preto, SP — Rua dos Aliados, 155, Campos Eliseos/ Tel. +55 (016) 628-1533
Rio de Janeiro, RJ — Rua Barao da Torre, 199, apt. 102, Ipanema/ Tel. +55 (021) 267-0052
Salvador, BA — Rua Alvaro Adorno, 17, Brotas/ Tel. +55 (071) 382-1064
Santos, SP — Rua Nabuco de Araujo, 151, Embare/ Tel. +55 (0132) 38-4655
São Carlos, SP — Rua Emilio Ribas, 195
São Paulo, SP — Av. Angelica, 2583/Tel. +55 (011) 259-7352
São Paulo, SP — Rua Otavio Tarquino de Souza, 299, Congonhas/ Tel. +55 (011) 536-4010

FARM COMMUNITIES

Autazes, AM — Nova Jarikandha/ Tel. +55 (092) 232-0202
Caruaru, PE — Nova Vrajadhama, Distrito de Murici, CP 283, CEP 55000-000
Curitiba, PR — Nova Goloka, Planta Carla, Pinhais

Parati, RJ — Goura Vrindavan, Bairro de Grauna, CP 062, CEP 23970-000
Pindamonhangaba, SP — Nova Gokula, Bairro Ribeiro Grande, CP 108, CEP 12400-000/ Tel. +55 (012) 982-9036
Teresopolis, RJ — Vrajabhumi, Canoas, CP 92687, CEP 25951-970

MEXICO

Guadalajara — Pedro Moreno No. 1791, Sector Juarez/ Tel. +52 (38) 160775
Mexico City — Gob. Tiburcio Montiel No. 45, 11850 Mexico, D.F./ Tel. +52 (5) 271-22-23
Saltillo — Blvd. Saltillo No. 520, Col. Buenos Aires

FARM COMMUNITY

Guadalajara — Contact ISKCON Guadalajara

ADDITIONAL RESTAURANTS

Orizaba — Restaurante Radhe, Sur 5 No. 50, Orizaba, Ver./ Tel. +52 (272) 5-75-25

PERU

Lima — Pasaje Solea 101 Santa Maria-Chosica/ Tel. +51 (014) 910891
Lima — Schell 634 Mira•ores
Lima — Av. Garcilazo de la Vega 1670-1680/ Tel. +51 (014) 259523

FARM COMMUNITY

Correo De Bella Vista — DPTO De San Martin

ADDITIONAL RESTAURANT

Cuzco — Espaderos 128

OTHER COUNTRIES

Asunción, Paraguay — Centro Bhaktivedanta, Mariano R. Alonso 925, Asunción/ Tel. +595 (021) 480-266
Bogotá, Colombia — Calle 72, nro.20-60, Bogota (mail: Apartado Aereo 58680, Zona 2, Chapinero)/ Tel. & Fax +57 (01) 2554529, 2482234
Buenos Aires, Argentina — Centro Bhaktivedanta, Andonaegui 2054 (1431)/ Tel. +54 (01) 521- 5567, 523-4232
Cali, Colombia — Avenida 2 EN, #24N-39/ Tel. +57 (023) 68-88-53
Caracas, Venezuela — Avenida Berlin, Quinta Tia Lola, La California Norte/ Tel. +58 (02) 225463
Chinandega, Nicaragua — Edificio Hare Krsna No. 108, Del Banco Nacional 10 mts. abajo/ Tel. +505 (341) 2359
Cochabamba, Bolivia — Av. Heroinas E-0435 Apt. 3 (mail: P. O. Box 2070)/ Tel. & Fax +591 (042) 54346
Essequibo Coast, Guyana — New Navadvipa Dham, Mainstay, Essequibo Coast
Georgetown, Guyana — 24 Uitvlugt Front, West Coast Demerara
Guatemala, Guatemala — Apartado Postal 1534
Guayaquil, Ecuador — 6 de Marzo 226 or V. M. Rendon/ Tel. +593 (04) 308412 y 309420
Managua, Nicaragua — Residencial Bolonia, De Galeria los Pipitos 75 mts. norte (mail: P.O. Box 772)/ Tel. +505 242759
Mar del Plata, Argentina — Dorrego 4019 (7600) Mar del Plata/ Tel. +54 (023) 745688
Montevideo, Uruguay — Centro de Bhakti-Yoga, Mariano Moreno 2660, Montevideo/ Tel. +598 (02) 477919
Panama, Republic of Panama — Via las Cumbres, entrada Villa Zaita, frente a INPSA No.1 (mail: P.O. Box 6-29-54, Panama)
Pereira, Colombia — Carrera 5a, #19-36
Quito, Ecuador — Inglaterra y Amazonas
Rosario, Argentina — Centro de Bhakti-Yoga, Paraguay 556, (2000) Rosario/ Tel. +54 (041) 252630, 264243
San José, Costa Rica — Centro Cultural Govinda, Av. 7, Calles 1 y 3, 235 mtrs. norte del Banco Anglo, San Pedro (mail: Apdo. 166,1002)/ Tel. +5206 23-52 38
San Salvador, El Salvador — Avenida Universitaria 1132, Media Quadra al sur de la Embajada Americana (mail: P.O. Box 1506)/ Tel. +503 25-96-17
Santiago, Chile — Carrera 330/ Tel. +56 (02) 698-8044
Santo Domingo, Dominican Republic — Calle Cayetano Rodriquez No. 254/ Tel. (809) 686-5665
Trinidad and Tobago, West Indies — Orion Drive, Debe/ Tel. +1 (809) 647-3165
Trinidad and Tobago, West Indies — Prabhupada Ave. Longdenville, Chaguanas

FARM COMMUNITIES

Argentina (Bhaktilata Puri) — Casilla de Correo No 77, 1727 Marcos Paz, Pcia. Bs. As., Republica Argentina
Bolivia — Contact ISKCON Cochabamba
Colombia (Nueva Mathura) — Cruzero del Guali, Municipio de Caloto, Valle del Cauca/ Tel. 612688 en Cali
Costa Rica — Nueva Goloka Vrindavana, Carretera a Paraiso, de la entrada del Jardin Lancaster (por Calle Concava), 200 metros al sur (mano derecha) Cartago (mail: Apdo. 166, 1002)/ Tel. +506 551-6752
Ecuador (Nueva Mayapur) — Ayampe (near Guayaquil)
Ecuador (Giridharidesha) — Chordeleg (near Cuenca), Cassiga Postal 01.05.1811, Cuenca/ Tel. +593 (7) 255735
El Salvador — Carretera a Santa Ana, Km. 34, Canton Los Indios, Zapotitan, Dpto. de La Libertad
Guyana — Seawell Village, Corentyne, East Berbice

ADDITIONAL RESTAURANTS

Buenos Aires, Argentina — Gusto Superior, Blanco Encalada 2722, 1428 Buenos Aires Cap. Fed./ Tel. +54 (01) 788 3023
Cochabamba, Bolivia — Gopal Restaurant, calle España N-0250 (Galeria Olimpia) (mail: P. O. Box 2070, Cochabamba)/ Tel. +591 (042) 26626
Guatemala, Guatemala — Callejor Santandes a una cuadra abajo de Guatel, Panajachel Solola
San Salvador, El Salvador — 25 Avenida Norte 1132
Santa Cruz, Bolivia — Snack Govinda, Av. Argomosa (1ero anillo), esq. Bolivar/ Tel. +591 (03) 345189

BHAGAVAD-GĪTĀ AS IT IS

The world's most popular edition of a timeless classic.

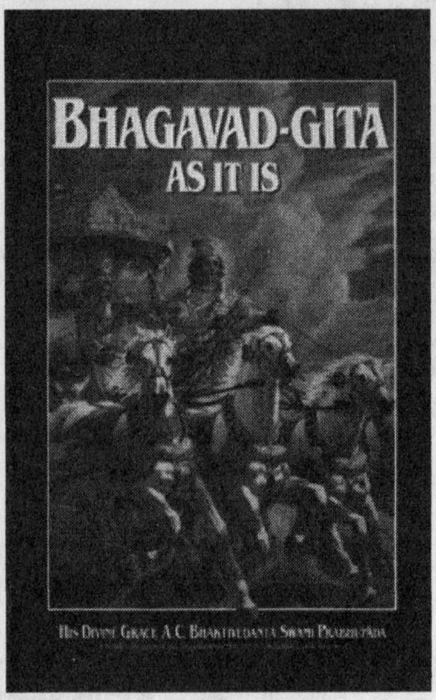

Throughout the ages, the world's greatest minds have turned to the *Bhagavad-gītā* for answers to life's perennial questions. Renowned as the jewel of India's spiritual wisdom, the *Gītā* summarizes the profound Vedic knowledge concerning man's essential nature, his environment, and ultimately his relationship with God. With more than fifty million copies sold in twenty languages, *Bhagavad-gītā As It Is,* by His Divine Grace A.C. Bhaktivedanta Swami Prabhupāda, is the most widely read edition of the *Gītā* in the world. It includes the original Sanskrit text, phonetic transliterations, word-for-word meanings, translation, elaborate commentary, and many full-color illustrations. (Pocket version: translation and commentary only.)

Pocket	Vinyl	Hard	Deluxe
$4.50	$8.50	$9.95	$19.95
BGS	BGV	BGH	BGD

ORDER TOLL FREE 1-800-927-4152

GREAT

VEGETARIAN DISHES

Featuring over 100 stunning full-color photos, this book is for spiritually aware people who want the exquisite taste of Hare Krishna cooking without a lot of time in the kitchen. The 240 international recipes were tested and refined by the author, world-famous Hare Krishna chef Kūrma dāsa.

240 recipes, 192 pages, coffee-table-size hardback

US: $19.95 #GVD

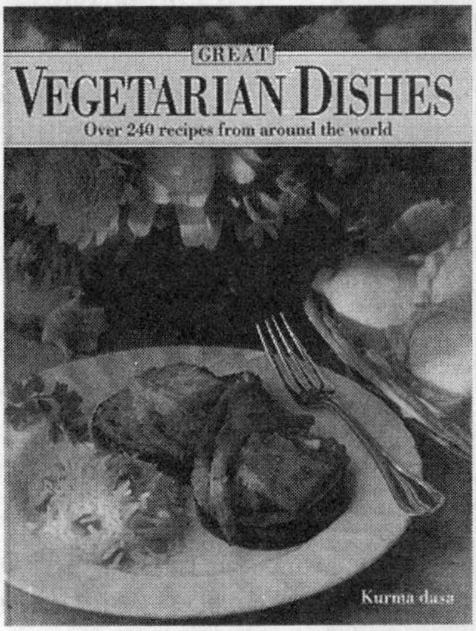

THE HARE KRISHNA BOOK OF

VEGETARIAN COOKING

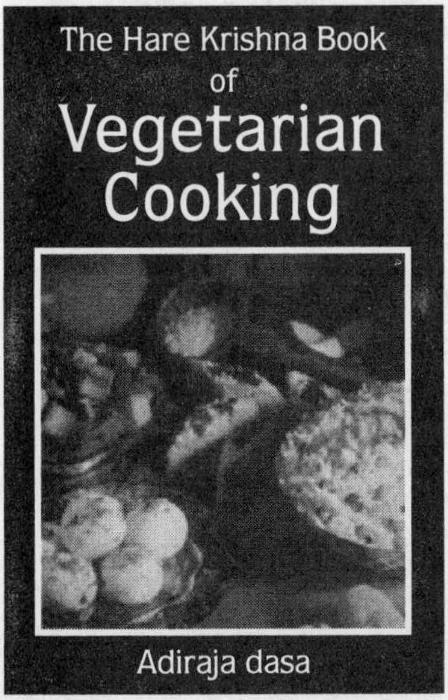

This colorfully illustrated, practical cookbook by Ādirāja dāsa not only helps you prepare authentic Indian dishes at home but also teaches you about the ancient tradition behind India's world-famous vegetarian cuisine.

130 kitchen-tested recipes, 300 pages, hardback

US: $11.50 #HKVC

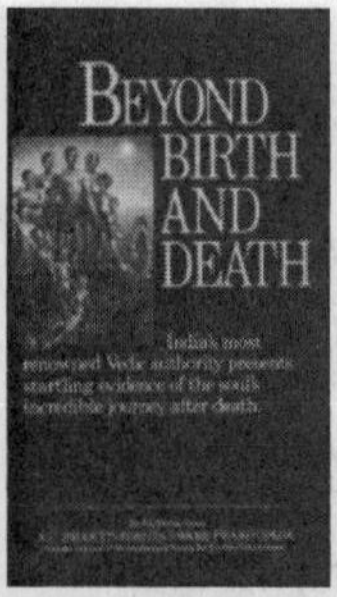

BEYOND BIRTH AND DEATH

What's the self? Can it exist apart from the physical body? If so, what happens to the self at the time of death? What about reincarnation? Liberation? In *Beyond Birth and Death* Śrīla Prabhupāda answers these intriguing questions and more.

Softbound, 96 pages

US$1.00 #BBD

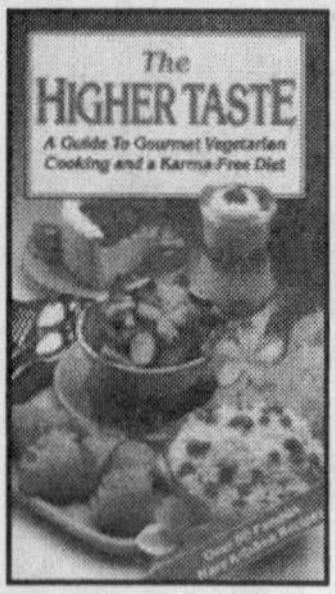

THE HIGHER TASTE

A Guide to Gourmet Vegetarian Cooking and a Karma-Free Diet

Illustrated profusely with black-and-white drawings and eight full-color plates, this popular volume contains over 60 tried and tested international recipes, together with the why's and how's of the Krishna conscious vegetarian life-style.

Softbound, 176 pages

US$1.50 #HT

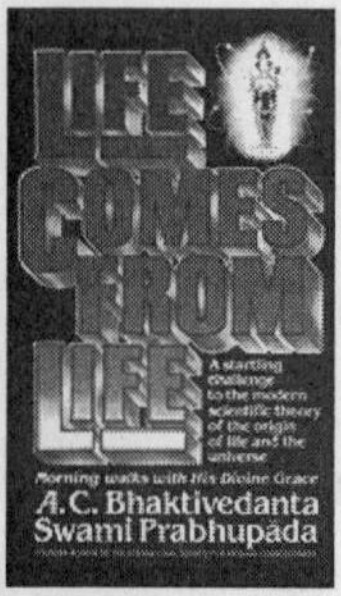

LIFE COMES FROM LIFE

In this historic series of talks with his disciples, Śrīla Prabhupāda uncovers the hidden and blatantly unfounded assumptions that underlie currently fashionable doctrines concerning the origins and purpose of life.

Softbound, 96 pages

US$1.50 #LCFL

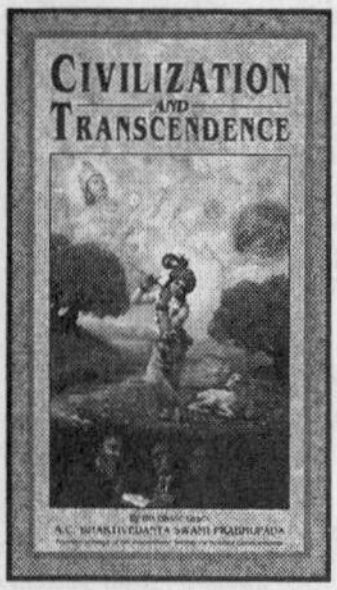

CIVILIZATION AND TRANSCENDENCE

In this book Śrīla Prabhupāda calls the bluff of modern materialistic culture: "Modern so-called civilization is simply a dog's race. The dog is running on four legs, and modern people are running on four wheels. The learned, astute person will use this life to gain what he has missed in countless prior lives—namely, realization of self and realization of God."

Softbound, 90 pages

US$1.00 #CT

Order Form

Make check or money order payable to The Bhaktivedanta Book Trust and send to:

The Bhaktivedanta Book Trust
Dept. QFE-H
3764 Watseka Avenue • Los Angeles, CA 90034

Name ____
Please Print

Address ____

City ______________________ ST _____ Zip ______________

Code	Description	Qty.	Price	Total

Subtotal US $ ____________

CA Sales Tax 8.25% US $ ____________

Shipping 15% of Subtotal (minimum $2.00) US $ ____________

TOTAL US $ ____________

To Place a Credit Card Order Please Call

1-800-927-4152

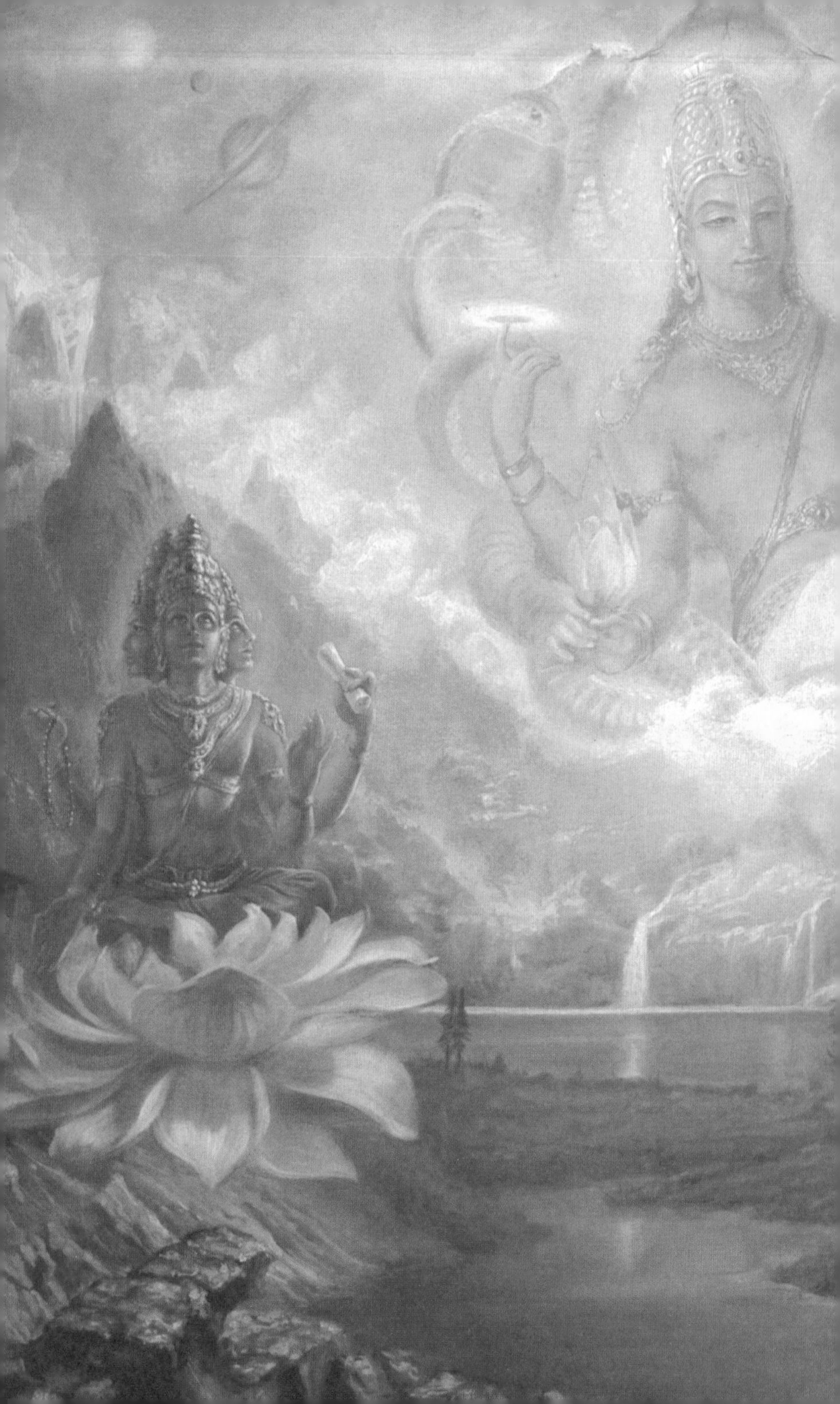